O.P.

GAY STUDIES

Sexual Differentiation of the Brain

Sexual Differentiation of the Brain

Based on a Work Session
of the Neurosciences Research Program

Robert W. Goy and Bruce S. McEwen

The MIT Press
Cambridge, Massachusetts, and London, England

This volume, based on an NRP Work Session held May 22–24, 1977, reflects the collaborative interaction, reviewing, and updating of the report by the participants prior to publication.

The Neurosciences Research Program, a research center of the Massachusetts Institute of Technology, is an interdisciplinary, interuniversity organization with the primary goal of facilitating the investigation of how the nervous system mediates behavior including the mental processes of man. To this end, the NRP, as one of its activities, conducts scientific meetings to explore crucial problems in the neurosciences and publishes reports of these Work Sessions. NRP is supported in part through Massachusetts Institute of Technology by National Institute of Mental Health Grant No. MH23132, National Institute of Neurological and Communicative Disorders and Stroke Contract No. NO1-NS-6-2343, National Science Foundation, The Grant Foundation, Max-Planck-Gesellschaft, Surdna Foundation, and through the Neurosciences Research Foundation, by The Arthur Vining Davis Foundations, The Herbert and Junia Doan Foundation, The Rogosin Foundation, The Alfred P. Sloan Foundation, van Ameringen Foundation, Inc., and Vollmer Foundation, Inc.

This book was printed and bound in the United States of America.

Library of Congress Cataloging in Publication Data
Main entry under title:

Sexual differentiation of the brain.

"Based on an NRP work session held May 22–24, 1977."
Bibliography: p. 158
Includes index.
1. Brain—Congresses. 2. Sex differences (Psychology)—Congresses. 3. Sexual behavior in animals—Congresses. 4. Sexual dimorphism (Animals)—Congresses. 5. Hormones, Sex—Physiological effect—Congresses. I. Goy, Robert W. II. McEwen, Bruce S. III. Neurosciences Research Program.
QP376.S435 599'.01'88 79-26288
ISBN 0-262-07077-4

CONTENTS

PARTICIPANTS

Susan W. Baker
Department of Psychiatry
Montefiore Hospital and Medical Center
Bronx, NY 10467

William W. Beatty
Department of Psychology
North Dakota State University
Fargo, ND 58102

John Czaja
Wisconsin Regional Primate Research Center
University of Wisconsin
Madison, WI 53706

Günter Dörner
Institut für Experimentelle Endokrinologie
Bereich Medizin der Humboldt-Universität zu Berlin
Berlin, German Democratic Republic

Anke A. Ehrhardt
Division of Child Psychiatry
New York State Psychiatric Institute
New York, NY 10032

Thomas O. Fox
Department of Neuroscience
Children's Hospital Medical Center
Boston, MA 02115

Arnold A. Gerall
Department of Psychology
Tulane University
New Orleans, LA 70118

Roger A. Gorski
Department of Anatomy
University of California School of Medicine
The Center for the Health Sciences
Los Angeles, CA 90024

Robert W. Goy
Wisconsin Regional Primate Research Center
University of Wisconsin
Madison, WI 53706

William T. Greenough
Department of Psychology
University of Illinois at Urbana-Champaign
Champaign, IL 61820

Ivan Lieberburg
The Rockefeller University
New York, NY 10021

Aubrey Manning
Department of Zoology
University of Edinburgh
Edinburgh, EH9, 3JT, Scotland

Bruce S. McEwen
Department of Neurobiology
The Rockefeller University
New York, NY 10021

Fernando Nottebohm
Field Research Center
The Rockefeller University
Millbrook, NY 12545

Alice S. Rossi
Department of Sociology
University of Massachusetts
Amherst, MA 01002

Francis O. Schmitt
Neurosciences Research Program
Jamaica Plain, MA 02130

C. Dominique Toran-Allerand
International Institute for Study of Human Reproduction
Columbia University
College of Physicians and Surgeons
New York, NY 10032

Judith Weisz
Division of Reproductive Biology
Hershey Medical Center
Hershey, PA 17033

Jean D. Wilson
Department of Internal Medicine
University of Texas
Southwestern Medical School
Dallas, TX 75235

Frederic G. Worden
Neurosciences Research Program
Jamaica Plain, MA 02130

Sexual Differentiation of the Brain

I. SEXUALLY DIMORPHIC BEHAVIOR: DEFINITION AND THE ORGANIZATIONAL HYPOTHESIS

Introduction

Sex differences in behavior, like sex differences in body structure, are determined by a combination of genetic, hormonal, and external environmental factors. Dissection of the relative importance of these factors has occupied a major part of the research and writing on the subject, and a discussion of these issues took much of the time during the Work Session. First, the term *sexually dimorphic* was discussed, after which the organizational hypothesis concerning the development of these behaviors in mammals and birds was outlined.

The term *dimorphism* refers to the existence of two distinct *forms* within a single species. The term sexually dimorphic behavior, by extension, implies two different forms of behavior exhibited by the male and the female. Some workers have accepted usage of the term to mean not two different forms of behavior, but a response shown exclusively by one sex and not by the other. While some behaviors observed under natural circumstances, e.g., the ejaculatory pattern, are present in one sex but not in the other of most species, few other kinds of behavior could be classified as sexually dimorphic by this strict definition. Under appropriate conditions of hormonal treatment and testing, for example, male rats will display receptive and lordosis behaviors, and female rats will exhibit circling and mounting behaviors. In the discussion and presentations that follow, the term sexually dimorphic does not usually indicate the presence of a given response in one sex exclusively and its absence in the other, but, rather, any measurable difference in the parameters of the response for the two sexes. Thus, for example, both males and females eat the same food, but one sex may ingest measurably more than the other, or one may eat more often than the other without actually eating more food. The running activity of rats provides a different kind of example. Both sexes run, but the temporal patterning of their locomotor activity, measured daily, is distinctly different. Again, in a given species, hypothetically at least, males and females may not differ in the amount of aggression shown, but may differ markedly with respect to the occasions or stimulus situations that evoke aggression. For example, in territorial species, males may attack primarily intruder males, and females may attack primarily intruder females. Finally, for hormonally mediated behavior, the sexes may differ only in the amount or kind of hormone normally involved in regulating the display of the behavior. Examples of such differences are to be found in the experimental induction of lordosis responses in male and female rodents when the male requires more estrogen than the female, or in the regulation of spontaneous mounting behavior, which, in some species, is facilitated by sequential estrogen and progesterone in the female and by testosterone in the male.

To describe these behavioral differences between the sexes as sexual dimorphisms does not violate common usage of the term by the morphological sciences. Among mammalian forms, both sexes have a pelvis. The difference between the sexes is not in the presence or absence of a pelvis or pelvic outlet, but in its size, girth, or other quantitative measure. Or there may be dynamic changes in the shape of the pelvis restricted to one sex and occasioned by pregnancy and parturition. Countless examples exist in morphology of sexual dimorphisms based only on quantitative differences, differences in intensity (e.g., coloration), or in response of a specific structure to hormonal stimulation. Nevertheless, despite the reasonableness of extending the term sexual dimorphism to behavioral differences, no implication is intended by the contributors concerning a structural or morphological basis for the measured dimorphism. The reader, moreover, is cautioned against drawing any such inference. Furthermore, the mere demonstration of sexual dimorphism cannot specify either its causation or its biological function. It was, in fact, the very task of the Work Session to determine, to the extent possible, the causes of a variety of described sexual dimorphisms in behavior, and for this purpose we have drawn heavily on the principles of sexual differentiation provided by embryologists, geneticists, and anatomists working with morphological sexual characteristics.

Current concepts of morphogenesis hold that the genetic sex of all vertebrates determines whether the embryonic genital ridge develops into a testis or an ovary. The means of action by which chromosomes direct the differentiation of the embryonic gonad are unknown; but it is known that the type of gonad differentiated determines by its secretory products whether male or female secondary reproductive organs develop. According to the organizational hypothesis (Phoenix et al., 1959), not only the reproductive organs but also the neural processes mediating sexual behavior in mammals have the intrinsic tendency to develop according to a female pattern of body structure and behavior. However, they pass through a restricted period when a bisexual potentiality exists in both sexes. Circulating androgens from the testes are both morphogenetic and psychogenetic. They enhance the development of male behavior, as well as the differentiation of male reproductive organs, and in both instances the modifications induced by the hormone are enduring. Up to this time, ovarian secretions have not been assigned a significant role in the differentiation of the sexual behavior or reproductive tract characteristics in mammals, and female sexual characters develop even in the complete absence of ovaries. For female behavior, the critical organizing influence seems, in fact, to be either the absence of potent androgens, or, alternatively, if they are present, their concentrations must be too low to initiate the events that lead to a masculine organization. Moreover, estrogens circulating in higher than normal concentrations not only do not promote the development of female characteristics, but in some mammalian species they may act like the androgens to enhance masculine behavioral traits. This "organizational" hypothesis addressed itself to hormones in the bloodstream and not in the cell. Information as to whether a specific androgen (e.g., like testosterone) is a prohormone that needs to be converted into another substance in the cytoplasm or nucleus of cells comprising target organs before it produces its enduring modifications is viewed as clarifying the cellular mechanism of organization rather than as contradictory to the hypothesis.

The hormonal induction of enduring effects on behaviors and morphology (i.e., the organizing action of the hormones) is restricted to a limited period of development, the so-called "critical period." Use of the "critical period" concept can be criticized on the grounds (1) that the changes induced by hormones are not identified physiologically and/or anatomically, and (2) that in the absence of such information the changes cannot be evaluated in terms of whether or not they are "critical." In preference to such loose usage of concepts, therefore, some investigators (Goy et al., 1964) have proposed the alternative term, "period of maximal susceptibility" (or sensitivity) to the actions of hormones on the tissues mediating behavior.

Regardless of the terminology, however, periods have been identified in early development when hormones can most readily effect enduring changes in the ways in which an individual is destined to behave. In placental mammals, this period of sensitivity for the developing offspring does not bear a constant relationship to the event of parturition or birth. Based strictly on empirical studies, the most effective period for modification is shortly after birth for the rat (Grady et al., 1965; Harris and Levine, 1965), the mouse (Campbell and McGill, 1970; Edwards, 1971), the hamster (Swanson, 1971), and the ferret (Baum, 1976); it is prior to birth for the guinea pig (Goy et al., 1964), the sheep (Short, 1974), and the rhesus monkey (Goy, 1966, 1968). In certain species, e.g., the dog (Beach and Kuehn, 1970; Beach et al., 1972), the relevant hormones may have to be present for some time both prior to and shortly following birth. In the few scattered studies that have been done with the rabbit, efforts to identify a maximally sensitive period have been unsuccessful. Campbell (1965) reported that a variety of steroids injected into female rabbits for a few days following birth failed to modify sexual behavior. Anderson (1970) reported that prenatal injections of androgen abolished maternal behavior of female rabbits but were without effect on adult sexual behavior, ovulation, or ability to maintain pregnancy. In view of demonstrated empirical precedents (e.g., dogs), it seems that the rabbit may also require exposure to appropriate steroids both pre- and post-natally in order to induce marked masculinization of genetic females. This problem needs to be reinvestigated.

For the limited number of species studied, there is an apparent relationship between fetal or larval opening of the eyes and the time of effective hormonal influence. In all cases, the developing organism has to be exposed to the hormone prior to eye-opening for enduring modifications to be induced. Since opening of the eye is correlated with neural maturation and development, it is relatively likely that hormones have to act on a nervous system at a specifiable stage of incomplete development in order to induce the changes of interest. While eye opening may, in a very general way, mark the end of the period of hormonal sensitivity, no specific event has been identified that serves as a marker for the beginning of this period. Considering, moreover, the extensive array of psychological functions, processes, and behavioral patterns now known to be influenced by hormones present during early stages of development, the utility of the notion of a single "period" should be questioned. Perhaps, rather, a sequence of "periods" exists, such that each step in the sequence is sensitive to organizational actions of the hormones on only one or a few specific traits. Some evidence supporting this possibility is presented in later sections of this report and, therefore, is not repeated here; but it may be of value to point out that the basic notion is consonant with what is known regarding the differentiation of separate portions of the mammalian male reproductive tract (Burns, 1961).

The original empirical studies on guinea pigs led to the hypothesis that androgens present before birth organized the pattern of sexual behavior into the male type (Phoenix et al., 1959). In those studies, evidence was presented demonstrating not only the enhancement of behavior normally typical of the male (mounting) but also suppression of behavior normally typical of the female (estrogen-progesterone induction of lordosis). Inasmuch as the male guinea pigs studied at the time showed only weak and irregular lordosis responses to induction procedures, such fragmentary responses were considered male-typical. Therefore, when the same kind of fragmentary and weak lordosis responses were found to be characteristic of genetic females exposed to androgen prenatally, this "suppressed" form of lordosis was conceptualized as one aspect of the masculinizing action of prenatal androgen. This suppressive action of lordosis was thought to be as significant to the organization of behavioral maleness as the enhancement of male behavior itself. In this respect, then, both suppression of female characters and enhancement of male characters were subsumed under "masculinization." In the time since the original statement of the organizational hypothesis, additional studies, some involving different species, have shown that the suppression of female-typical behavior can be accomplished independently of the enhancement of male-typical behavior. These discoveries have led to the adoption of a new terminology. The term "defeminization" has been adopted and widely used to refer to hormonal effects involving the suppression of female-typical behavior in genetic females only. The term "masculinization" is now generally reserved only for hormonal effects involving the enhancement of male-typical behaviors in genetic females. For the genetic male, complementary terms of "feminization" and "demasculinization" have been brought into usage. More complete discussion of these terminological problems can be found in Beach (1971) and Goy and Goldfoot (1973).

The real advantage of the use of terms like masculinization and defeminization (or feminization and demasculinization) lies not alone in the conceptualization of these as independent processes. The use of these terms encourages questions about spontaneous bisexuality that might be overlooked with a different theoretical framework. For example, some female guinea pigs show frequent mounting behavior as well as vigorous lordosis at the time of spontaneous or induced estrus, and these characteristics are genetically influenced (Goy and Young, 1957; Goy and Jakway, 1959). Adoption of the newer terminology readily facilitates the question: "What is the agent that masculinizes without defeminizing these females?" An alternative restatement of this question might be: "What are the conditions that impose a bisexual organization on females within a defined genome?" The summaries of discussions from the Work Session only hint at possible answers to such questions, but, at the very least, they show that the contemporary form of question avoids more of the purely semantic problems than was previously possible. While there is still reasonable and serious dispute regarding the biological cause of different organizations of sexuality and sexual behavior, hormonal hypotheses have earned a respectability that allows their inspection even for problems of human sexual behavior, a permission that was not readily granted by clinical workers a few decades ago.

As far as can be ascertained, behavioral traits that exhibit sexual dimorphism are influenced only by the gonadal hormones, regardless of whether these hormones are secreted by the gonads, the adrenals, or both. Restriction of behavioral sexual dimorphisms to gonadal hormone influence may reflect the fact that many or all of these traits are directly or indirectly related to reproductive fitness. As Nottebohm emphasizes in his discussion of avian sexual dimorphisms in a later section of this report, the functions of behavioral dimorphisms in attraction and arousal of mating partners are adaptive when their display reflects full reproductive competence (i.e., fully functional gonads).

Studies of sexually dimorphic behavior are numerous for mammalian species and much less well represented for other forms. It will not be surprising, therefore, if what has been learned about hormonal influences on such characters requires revision and extension as more data become available. Even for mammals, however, evidence clearly supports the classification of male-typical characters into three basic types in terms of their relations to the gonadal hormones. Type I encompasses those behavioral characteristics that cannot be brought to full expression unless the relevant hormone(s) is (are) present in adequate amounts in the circulation during both the critical period of early development and *also* during a later life stage. Some behavioral traits, in other words, require both early organizational actions and later activational actions of the hormones. It is not without interest, moreover, that the hormones that accomplish the organizational effects and those that activate the behavior at a later age are most often the same. Examples of behavioral traits that require hormonal actions both early and late in development are male intromissive and ejaculatory behavior (see Gerall's section) and the male fighting behavior of some strains of mice (see Beatty's section). These behavioral traits find a distinct parallel in the actions of androgens on male accessory reproductive organs like the prostate and seminal vesicles. For these structures, organizational actions during an early critical period first effect structural differentiation, and later in life activational actions induce secretory function.

A second type of relationship (Type II) characterizes those behaviors that seemingly require only activation at later ages by the appropriate hormone. For these behavioral traits either androgen is not necessary during the early critical period, or the amount of androgen normally present at that time in both sexes is sufficient for their organization. An example of this kind of trait is the yawning behavior of rhesus monkeys (Goy and Resko, 1972). This response is ordinarily displayed much more frequently by adult males than by females or juveniles of either sex (Bielert, 1978). However, its frequency of display by females or juveniles can be augmented to a level equal to or exceeding that of the normal male by administration of exogenous testosterone. The mounting behavior of some strains of rats may be another example (Whalen et al., 1969), although females that mount as adults due to exogenous testosterone may have undergone some in utero virilization by exposure to their brothers' androgens (Clemens and Coniglio, 1971). Morphological parallels exist for this type of trait as well, and the induction of the growth of facial hair and balding response of human beings are well-known examples. These traits, more common in adult males than females, can be induced in the latter by exogenous testosterone given only in adulthood.

Type II behavioral traits, which can be activated at will independently of organizational influences, are not enduring features of the individual. Such traits are manifested only during the time the activational hormone is present. When the hormone is removed by castration or declines spontaneously, the manifestation of the behavior is measurably altered, usually lessened in frequency or intensity. These traits depend entirely on concurrent hormonal levels during later ages when the behavior is normally displayed, and they differ from Type I traits not in their activational requirements but in their independence from organizational influences of the hormones during the critical period.

Type III traits, perhaps because of their more recent discovery, or perhaps because definitive evidence for them is more difficult to obtain, occur less frequently than Types I and II. These behavioral traits require only organizational actions of androgens, and no activational influence is required for their full expression by the individual. Such traits are manifested as well, or nearly as well, in males castrated prior to puberty (but after the end of the early critical period) as in intact males. They cannot be "activated" in spayed females by administration of exogenous androgen during the postcritical period stage of development; but they can be easily induced in females by appropriate treatment with androgens during the critical period. Examples of such types of behavior are the juvenile play and mounting behavior of rhesus monkeys (see later discussion by Goy in this section) and the micturitional patterns of the dog (Martins and Valle, 1948; Beach, 1974). No parallel morphological systems come readily to mind beyond the basic sexual differentiation of the reproductive tract tissues.

Recognition of the general and usual existence of these three types of relationships between hormones and sexually dimorphic behavior provides a perspective that renders a common mechanism of hormonal action unlikely. The complete contrast between Type II and Type III, the former operating entirely through activational mechanisms and the latter entirely through organizational mechanisms, suggests, at the very least, that the nature of the hormonal interactions with cellular machinery might contrast correspondingly.

This introduction to the problems of hormonal regulation of behavioral sexual dimorphism would be incomplete without some added information on other vertebrate classes. Birds, reptiles, amphibians, and fishes are clearly more diversified and less completely studied than mammals. In one precocial avian species, the Japanese quail, Adkins (1975) has shown that injection of fertile eggs on day 10 of incubation with either testosterone propionate or estradiol benzoate produced feminized males and normal females. Such treated males showed suppression of male sexual responses as adults and augmentation of feminine receptivity, exactly the opposite of the general effects of steroid treatment in mammals. Estradiol was clearly more potent in demasculinization and feminization than testosterone, and the latter hormone probably accomplishes its organizational effects through aromatization to estradiol or estrone. Thus, although organizational influences of hormones are demonstrable in birds, both the effective hormone and the sex affected are different from the mammalian case, and resolution of this difference has been sought in terms of the influence of heterogamety on hormonal organization. Paralleling the mammalian story, however, the period for organizing actions of estrogens in birds is prenatal in precocial and postnatal in altricial forms. Orcutt (1971), using altricial pigeons, obtained evidence for demasculinization and feminization of males treated with implants of estradiol for varying periods of time post-hatching.

Studies appropriate to the concerns of the Work Session have not been carried out in reptiles, and the information on amphibians and fishes is incomplete for present purposes. Nevertheless, frogs, toads, newts, and salamanders can be completely sex-reversed by incubating fertilized eggs in water containing small amounts of hormone (Burns, 1961; Foote, 1964; Gallien, 1965, 1967). These sex reversals are so complete that genetic females grown in water containing testosterone develop fully functional testes, produce sperm, and mate with normal females to produce only female offspring. Conversely, in other species, males grown in water containing small amounts of estradiol are comparably reversed and will mate with normal males. Unfortunately, for these species information is lacking on specific hormone-behavior relationships in adults and on the reversibility of sexually dimorphic behavior at later ages. In short, it is not known whether critical periods exist for the organization of sexually dimorphic behaviors of any sort.

Of all the vertebrate phyla, fishes are the most diversified and least understood. Among teleosts, hermaphroditism is an extremely common occurrence. However, our search for examples that might provide evidence for organizational influences that conform to those of mammals has to exclude these spontaneously hermaphroditic forms. Complete transformation of all female offspring into males has been accomplished in *Tilapia mossambica* by treating fry with methyltestosterone for about 2 months after hatching (Clemens and Inslee, 1968). Newly hatched goldfish, treated for about the same period of time post-hatching, were transformed either to all-female broods when estrogens were used or to all-male broods when androgens were used (Yamamoto and Kajishima, 1968). The addition of either testosterone or estradiol to the aquarium water of young cichlids resulted in feminization of males, and such feminized males could be bred to normal males (Hackmann and Reinboth, 1974). When sexual differentiation of the gonad normally occurs before birth (or hatching), treatment of fry is ineffective. For the viviparous guppy, treatment of gravid females with methyltestosterone for only 24 hours resulted in all-male broods (Dzwillo, 1962).

In general these studies of experimental sex reversal have not investigated hormonal influences at later ages, and the extent to which these same species could be sex-reversed as adults has not been carefully worked out. A loss of plasticity with maturity is certain for hormonal reversal of the gonad in some forms (Hackmann and Reinboth, 1974) and is suggested for behavior by the finding that adult female *Platypoecilus variatus* treated with methyltestosterone showed only weak and preliminary male courtship patterns (Laskowski (1953). Clearly, much more work is needed before concepts like the critical period can be meaningfully applied to fishes, and for spontaneously reversing forms such a concept is not likely ever to be applicable without modification.

Spontaneous sex reversal from functional female to functional male is well known and occurs among such diverse forms as zooplanktivores (Popper and Fishelson, 1973), cleaner wrasses (Robertson, 1972), gobies (Lassig, 1977), and parrot fish (Choat and Robertson, 1975). Though "spontaneous," once reversal has occurred, no reversal or regression to the original type has been documented for any species. Recently, Shapiro (1977) has completed an elegantly detailed study of sex reversal in the protogynous coral reef fish, *Anthias squamipinnis.* In this species all juveniles mature as females, and only some transform later into males. This social species lives in heterosexual groups, and the loss of a single male from the group is followed by a surprisingly rapid sex reversal (requiring only 1 week or so) in one of the females. The changes include transformation to the color pattern, gonadal histology, and behavior of the normal male. For each group, the transformation is limited to a single female, and the factors determining which female will undergo tranformation are not entirely clear. In part, however, the transforming female is suddenly treated (i.e., behaved toward) quite differently by the other female members of the group. Well in advance of any outward physical signs of change, the nonreversing females behave toward the reversing female as though she were male. Shapiro (1977) argues that, since all-female groups occur in nature, it is the change in social behavioral patterns that are more causal to the females' sex reversal than the removal or loss of a male. This fascinating model for social environmental control of hormonal functions deserves detailed future study. The phenomenon may have parallels or even partial homologies at other phyletic levels. The opposite type of spontaneous sex reversal (from male to female) also occurs among fishes. In the anemone fish *Amphiprion,* a monogamous but group-living form, the single female (always the largest and oldest in the group) suppresses the transformation from male to female by aggressive dominance over the smaller and subordinate males (Fricke and Fricke, 1977). Only one of the males in the group, the most dominant, has fully functional testes, and in all other males testicular development is correlated with dominance status.

This brief survey of vertebrate sexuality serves only to show that no fundamental uniformity exists that is readily apparent. Phyla differ, as do species within phyla, with regard (1) to the hormone that has morphogenetic and psychogenetic potential, (2) to the genetic sex that can be more easily reversed, (3) to the state of maturation at which reversal can occur, (4) to the extent to which sex can be hormonally reversed, and (5) with regard (probably) to the role of hormones in the organization and activation of specific behaviors. Nevertheless, despite these differences, there is, as yet, no compelling evidence against the most abstract level of generalization that would assert the possibility that both organizational and activational influences of the gonadal hormones are represented among all vertebrate phyla. The fact that both kinds of hormonal influence may not be demonstrable in every species is not, after all, a more difficult conceptual flaw than the circumstance that both influences are not always demonstrable for every type of sexually dimorphic behavior shown by a single species. Nor is it any more disconcerting, logically, than the fact that a sexual dimorphism found in one species may not be present in another, or may be present but totally reversed in a third. On the contrary, the boundless variation of behavioral and morphological sexual dimorphisms is one of the richest challenges to empirical science in general and to endocrinology and neurology in particular. In searching out mechanisms of proximate causation, we cannot afford to ignore the adaptive functions of these dimorphisms; we must be willing to entertain the possibility that some dimorphisms have neither a genetic nor a hormonal basis. The notion that selection strongly favors the complete environmental determination of sex in some species (Charnov and Bull, 1977) obliges us to tolerate a possible like determination of behavioral characters typical to each sex. For some highly social species, like the human being, culture may define the types and limits of sexual dimorphisms. Worse luck yet, the individual human being may be forced to learn or acquire those dimorphisms that, like the sex-reversing *Anthias squamipinnis,* the behavior of his or her peers thrusts upon him/her.

II. SEX DIFFERENCES IN BEHAVIOR: RODENTS, BIRDS, AND PRIMATES

Differentiation of Sexual Behavior in Rodents

Gerall provided the Work Session with an extensive background, citing many experiments demonstrating that, when fetal or altricial mammals are exposed to certain steroid hormones, they will, as adults, display heterotypical sexual behavior with higher frequency and quality than untreated subjects. Thus, the organizational action of perinatal hormones has most often been viewed as modifying the threshold of elicitation of mating and other behaviors involved in reproduction, including aggression and maternal activities. The nature of these behaviors and the degree to which they are restricted to one sex or are shared by each sex vary considerably among species. Thus, at this stage of knowledge, it has been necessary to test the implications of the organizational hypothesis with more than one species. Perinatal hormone manipulations have not yielded the same results in different species, although species differences in alteration of sexual behavior after perinatal administration of androgens to females differ primarily in degree, not in direction. The results for a wide variety of mammalian species are summarized in Table 1. These discrepant findings have been instructive in directing attention to physiological or other variables that must be included in a general theory attempting to understand the ontogeny of reproductive behavior.

The two most frequently studied rodents are the rat and hamster. The receptivity pattern of the rat includes soliciting or proceptive behaviors (Beach, 1976), including darting, hopping, and ear wiggling, which precede and perhaps determine the occurrence of mounting by the male. The lordosis, which occurs only when skin is contacted, is relatively brief, generally lasting while the male is mounting and 1 or 2 seconds thereafter. Proceptive behaviors are not evident in the receptive hamster, and her lordosis, once assumed, is often held for longer than 5 min. Its maintenance is considerably less dependent on contact than it is in the rat. During a mating test, the male hamster not only engages in fewer preliminary behaviors but mounts less frequently than the male rat.

A consistent difference also exists between these species: the tendency to exhibit heterotypical sexual behaviors. Male hamsters more

TABLE 1

Effects of Perinatal Administration of Androgen to Females on the Development of Sexually Dimorphic Traits [Gerall]

Species	Critical* period	Dimorphic Characteristic†			Reference
		Ovulation	Type of sexual behavior		
			Female	Male	
Rat	Post	↓↓↓↓	↓↓↓	↑	See text
Mouse	Post	↓↓↓↓	↓↓↓	↑↑	Barraclough and Leathem, 1954 Edwards and Burge, 1971
Hamster	Post	↓	↓	↑↑↑↑	Carter et al., 1972; Paup et al., 1972, 1974; Whitsett and Vandenbergh, 1975
Ferret	Post	?	0	↑↑↑	Baum, 1976
Dog	Pre + post	?	↓↓	↑↑	Beach and Kuehn, 1970; Beach et al., 1972
Guinea pig	Pre	↓↓	↓↓↓	↑↑	Phoenix et al., 1959; Goy et al., 1964; Brown-Grant and Sherwood, 1971
Sheep	Pre	↓↓	↓↓	↑↑	Short, 1974; Clarke et al., 1976b
Rhesus	Pre	Onset delayed	?	↑↑	Goy, 1970a,b

*Pre = prenatal; post = postnatal.
†Arrows indicate direction and relative ease of obtaining effect: ↓ = defeminization; ↑ = masculinization; 0 = no effect.

readily display female behaviors than male rats, and female rats more readily manifest male behaviors than female hamsters. Lordosis is induced by estradiol and progesterone treatment of male hamsters castrated as adults (Tiefer, 1970). A similar treatment does not induce lordosis in adult male rats. Mounting occurs spontaneously in neonatally untreated intact female rats but rarely in intact female hamsters. Administration of testosterone propionate (TP) in oil readily induces mounting in ovariectomized rats but not in hamsters (Paup et al., 1972; Whitsett and Vandenbergh, 1975). Finally, a response resembling the ejaculatory pattern of males can be elicited from normal adult female rats by either prolonged estrogen treatment or by electrical stimulation in adulthood (Emery and Sachs, 1975). A similar behavior has not been observed in female hamsters.

The disparity between rat and hamster sexual behavior tendencies can be rationalized, at least in part, by arguing that hamsters are exposed to less androgen or are less responsive to circulating androgen during their critical periods of development. As a predictable consequence of either circumstance, the male hamster would have the lower threshold for lordosis and the female hamster a higher threshold for mounting than their rat counterparts.

In many rodents, a particularly important portion of the critical period for the organization of sexual processes occurs before birth. Clemens (1974) correlated the number of male rats in a litter with the propensity of the females in that litter to show mounting behavior when tested in adulthood. The probability of mounting was 0% in females from litters with 0 to 1 male, but 75% in females from litters with 4 to 5 males. Moreover, preliminary results indicated that both anogenital distance, a reliable measure of androgen exposure, and mounting behavior in adulthood were highest for females located in utero in closest proximity to males (Clemens and Coniglio, 1971). These parameters were the lowest for females located in utero distant to males. These studies, which were replicated in mice by Gandelman and co-workers (1977) and vom Saal and Bronson (1978), were extended in rats by Tobet, Dunlap, and Gerall,* who determined the sequential position of male and female fetuses by observing the birth of pups in unilaterally ovariectomized mothers. All of the females were injected with TP when 3 days old to induce sterility after puberty. The results showed that females located in utero between two males tended to have longer anogenital distances and to develop persistent estrus sooner than females situated between two females. The females, having resided between two males, mounted significantly more frequently in mating tests after administration of TP than females residing adjacent to females.

In addition, it is known that the male rat testis is active before birth and considerable androgen can be detected in both male and female fetuses (Resko et al., 1968; Turkelson et al., 1977). Observations such as these, together with reports that antiandrogen treatment of rats in utero results in significant blockage of masculinization (Ward

*S. Tobet, J.L. Dunlap, and A.A. Gerall: Influence of fetal position on neonatal androgen-induced sterility and on sexual behavior; MS in preparation.

and Renz, 1972), indicate that the critical period with respect to masculine development begins in the rat before birth.

The gestation period for the rat is 22 to 23 days, whereas it is only 16 days for the hamster. If the gonads were developing at roughly similar rates, then both male and female hamster fetuses would be exposed to considerably less testicular androgen than rat fetuses. Lack of androgen during the fetal period could account for subsequent diminution of tissue reactivity to androgen. Whether because of less exposure to fetal androgen or to intrinsic cellular causes, hamsters, in general, show less responsiveness to androgen than rats do. More androgen is required to suppress permanently both ovulation and lordosis behavior in female hamsters than in rats (Swanson, 1971; Noble, 1974; Whitsett and Vandenbergh, 1975). Whereas secretions from the postnatal testes diminish markedly the lordosis induced by estradiol benzoate and progresterone in adult male rats, they have much less inhibitory influence in hamsters (Swanson and Crossley, 1971). Also, it appears that more TP is required to restore sexual behavior in castrated male hamsters than in rats.

In general, data describing the degree to which normal and perinatally hormonally manipulated hamsters and rats manifest heterotypical mating behaviors can be considered as compatible with the organizational hypothesis. Also, differences between these heterotypical sexual tendencies can be encompassed, at least in part, by the hypothesis. However, whether the differing homotypical sexual responses of these same species can be explained is not clear. Are the fewer mounting responses shown by male hamsters in comparison to male rats and the longer duration of lordosis exhibited by female hamsters relative to female rats due to differences in amount or utilization of androgen during organization? While this might be an interesting and testable question, it is offered to emphasize a restriction of the organizational hypothesis. As stated, it is not intended to explain all sexual dimorphisms or species differences, or to generate experiments that can identify variables to eliminate these differences in behavior. Behavior depends not only on interrelations between the neuroendocrine system involved in reproductive processes but also on sensory and motor capabilities and morphological characteristics of each species. At first, the hypothesis should evolve principles describing how the efficacy of activating hormones for normally occurring homotypical and heterotypical behaviors in a given species would be altered by modifying its perinatal hormone environment. In mammals, it would be anticipated that the responsiveness to hormones typically activating normally occurring female behaviors would be reduced, while those activating normally occurring male behaviors would be enhanced by perinatal androgen. Generalizing across species becomes more feasible when significant structural or morphological differences can be identified and specified as significant variables. Differences in sensorimotor capabilities, in secondary sexual organ structure, and in neural complexity could play a role in how sexual dimorphisms are expressed and, hence, how they are activated by hormones. However, facilitation or activation of sexual behavior above a reference for that species in a given circumstance should be predictable by principles common to all species.

Morphological considerations have entered into all attempts to understand the mediation of sexually dimorphic behaviors. It has been argued that the effects of perinatal hormones on behavior can be better accounted for by changes in peripheral organs than by modification of the central nervous system (Beach, 1971). Since perinatally administered TP invariably causes the clitoris to hypertrophy and assume penile characteristics, it has been argued that increases in masculine behavior displayed by treated females could be attributed to this peripheral modification. Similarly, the decrease in male sexual behavior reliably recorded in neonatally castrated males could be due to impaired phallus development. Therefore, no changes in the central nervous system have to be assumed. Considerable data have been amassed recently to render this view less plausible than when originally proposed. Androgens other than testosterone have been injected that stimulate male phallus development without major effects on the central nervous system. Neonatally castrated male rats injected with fluoxymesterone have normal penises but do not exhibit normal sexual responses (Hart, 1972).

Thus, having a normally developed, adequate penis in itself does not insure normal sexual behavior. An androgen must be present that has specific effects on the central nervous system. Another line of evidence against a simple explanation based on peripheral site of action of perinatal androgen is that male-typical responses not dependent upon distinctive peripheral organs, such as aggression, have been shown to increase in females given testosterone propionate neonatally and to decrease in males having diminished neonatal androgen (Edwards, 1968; Bronson and Desjardins, 1970). Also, neonatal castration of male rats consistently leads to increased lordosis tendency; these males have no female secondary organs. However, despite such evidence against a complete determinative influence of peripheral structures, the expression of adequate sexual behavior clearly is partly dependent upon adequate peripheral structures. When observed, suppression of behavior must be carefully interpreted and assurances must be provided that it is not occurring because of modified or inadequate peripheral organs. It is doubtful that the peripheral-central controversy will ever be settled completely; but, at the present time, perhaps the most telling argument that perinatal hormones do not bring about their change in behavior solely by peripheral organ changes comes from current studies, such as those reported at the Work Session, directly correlating changes in neuronal structure with levels of perinatal hormones (Raisman and Field, 1973).

Attention has also been focused on the effect of perinatal hormone manipulation on the onset of puberty and on longevity of reproductive capabilities. In rats, neonatal administration of TP either has no effect or hastens the onset of puberty as measured by the date of vaginal opening (Barraclough, 1966). In hamsters, guinea pigs, and rhesus monkeys, perinatal androgen is associated with a marked delay in onset of puberty (Goy, 1970a; Brown-Grant and Sherwood, 1971). An explanation for these species differences is not available. Nor is it known whether perinatal androgen influences onset of puberty by altering ovarian secretion, timing in the brain, or somatic metabolic processes. Dose-dependent delays in the onset of puberty as measured by age of descent of testes and onset of adequate sexual behavior have been recorded in rats administered estradiol benzoate (EB) (Brown-Grant et al., 1975; Zadina, 1977). Similarly, large doses of androgen administered before the fifth day of age also delay puberty in male rats. The delay in puberty in male rats has been associated with retarded secretion of adequate amounts of follicle-stimulating hormone (FSH) (Brown-Grant et al., 1975).

A series of studies are being performed in Gerall's laboratory relating perinatal androgen treatment to longevity of estrous behavior (Gerall et al., 1979). The general finding is that perinatal androgen decreases the maximum level of lordosis responsiveness induced by dosages of activating hormone, which in most instances consists of EB and progesterone. The decrease in behavioral responsiveness is directly proportional to the amount of TP and inversely proportional to the age when administered neonatally. The rate of decline from this maximum level as a function of age is not accelerated by perinatal androgen. Longevity of reproductive behavior is shorter in perinatally androgenized females, primarily because they have a lower capacity to utilize hormones and therefore reach a threshold of nonresponding sooner than nontreated animals. In this manner, perinatal androgen may limit the response to activating hormones for the entire life of the animal.

Attempts to find a role for ovarian secretions during perinatal development have not met with notable success. When administered exogenously, most dosages of estrogen either have no effect or decrease the capacity of the female to exhibit receptive behaviors (Gerall et al., 1972a). Evidence that perinatal ovarian secretions might have an effect on sexually dimorphic behaviors has been reported by Blizard and Denef (1973) in rats. Also, perinatal ovarian secretion increases receptivity in neonatally androgenized female and neonatally castrated male rats (Farrell et al., 1977; Dunlap et al., 1978).

Sex Differences in Nonreproductive Behaviors In Rodents

Although the effects on nonreproductive behavior of manipulating gonadal hormones during the perinatal period have been much less thoroughly studied than the influence of similar manipulations on sexual behavior, it is clear that gonadal hormones can exert important organizational influences on many behaviors that are not related to reproduction in any obvious way. This fact is of such importance in assessing the relation of studies on rodents to studies of primates, including the human species, that it should be given special emphasis (see Beatty's summary of the relevant literature on this topic in Table 2). Before presentation of the details, however, some general comments that apply to the subject of sex differences in nonreproductive behavior are worth itemizing.

1. Sexual dimorphisms in these behaviors are usually expressed as differences in the *quality* of behavior exhibited under specified conditions.

2. For many nonreproductive behaviors, differences in genital morphology have no obvious relationship to performance.

3. For many nonreproductive behaviors, sex differences are small in magnitude and occur as differences in *average* performance

TABLE 2

Organizational and Activational Effects of Gonadal Hormones on Nonreproductive Behaviors in Rodents [Beatty]

Behavior	Evidence for organizational effect early in development	Reference	Evidence for activational effects	Reference
Activity				
Running wheel	+	Gerall et al., 1972a; Gentry and Wade, 1976b	++	Roy and Wade, 1975 (and many others)
Open-field	++	Gray et al., 1965; Swanson, 1966, 1967 Pfaff and Zigmond, 1971; Blizard and Denef, 1973; Bengelloun et al., 1976	+	Quadagno et al., 1972; Slater and Blizard, 1976
			–	Bronstein and Hirsch, 1974; Bengelloun et al., 1976
Aggression				
Shock-elicited (rat)	+	Conner et al., 1969; Powell et al., 1971	+	Hutchinson et al., 1965; Bernard and Paolino, 1975
Isolation-induced (mouse)	++	Bronson and Desjardins, 1968, 1970; Edwards, 1969	++	Beeman, 1947; Edwards, 1969; Erpino and Chappelle, 1973; Luttge and Hall, 1973a,b
Spontaneous (hamster)	?	Payne and Swanson, 1972c	++	Payne and Swanson, 1971a,b, 1972a,b

TABLE 2 (continued)

Organizational and Activational Effects of Gonadal Hormones on Nonreproductive Behaviors in Rodents [Beatty]

Behavior	Evidence for organizational effect early in development	Reference	Evidence for activational effects	Reference
Sensory factors				
Taste preferences	++	Valenstein et al., 1967; Wade and Zucker, 1969; Zucker, 1969; Zucker et al., 1972; Krecek, 1973; Shapiro and Goldman, 1973	+	Wade and Zucker, 1970a; Marks and Hobbs, 1972
			–	Hirsch and Bronstein, 1976
Reaction to shock	?	Beatty and Fessler, 1977a	+	Marks and Hobbs, 1972; Marks et al., 1972 Davis et al., 1976;
			–	Beatty and Beatty, 1970; Beatty and Fessler, 1977a
Feeding and body weight	++	Beatty et al., 1970; Bell and Zucker, 1971; Slob and van der Werff ten Bosch, 1975; Tarttelin et al., 1975; Dubuc, 1976; Wade, 1976	++	Zucker, 1972; Slob et al., 1973; Tarttelin and Gorski, 1973; Czaja and Goy, 1975; Gentry and Wade, 1976a; Roy and Wade, 1976; Wade, 1976

TABLE 2 (continued)

Organizational and Activational Effects of Gonadal Hormones on Nonreproductive Behaviors in Rodents [Beatty]

Behavior	Evidence for organizational effect early in development	Reference	Evidence for activational effects	Reference
Learning				
Active avoidance acquisition	+	Beatty and Beatty, 1970; Scouten, 1972; Scouten et al., 1975	–	Beatty and Beatty, 1970; Scouten et al., 1975
Active avoidance extinction	?		?	Ikard et al., 1972; Telegdy and Stark, 1973; Gray, 1977
Passive avoidance	?	Bengelloun et al., 1976	–	Bengelloun et al., 1976
DRL	?	Beatty et al., 1975a	+	Beatty, 1973a
Maze learning	+	Stewart et al., 1975	?	
Taste aversion	?		+	Chambers, 1976
Brain lesions				
Septal area	++	Phillips and Lieblich, 1972; Phillips and Deol, 1973 Lieblich et al., 1974 Bengelloun et al., 1976	–	Phillips and Lieblich, 1972; Bengelloun et al., 1976
Caudate and globus pallidus	?		+	Studelska and Beatty, 1978
Ventromedial hypothalamus	+	Valenstein, 1968	+	Valenstein et al., 1969

++ = Sufficient data to clearly establish an effect; + = data suggestive of an effect; – = data suggest absence of an effect· ? = no data or very incomplete data.

between groups. Sex differences in these behaviors are often markedly influenced by species, strain, and the testing conditions. Ostensibly trivial variations in experimental procedures can profoundly affect the magnitude of the average difference in performance.

4. While we are a very long way from understanding which constitutional and environmental variables are important, the available data suggesting how little we really know about such factors should, at least, lead us to reject, as premature, attempts to explain all sex differences in nonreproductive behavior in terms of unitary and global but typically loose constructs such as "emotionality," "perceptual and cognitive restructuring," "intelligence," or "energy level."

Running Wheel Activity

Sex differences in running wheel activity in the rat were described more than 50 years ago when it was also shown that castration reduced activity in both sexes as well as abolished the sex difference (e.g., Hitchcock, 1925). More recent work has shown that estrogen is clearly the activating hormone in males as well as females: testosterone injections merely provide a substrate for estrogen production (Roy and Wade, 1975), perhaps in the anterior hypothalamic-preoptic area where central estradiol benzoate implants stimulate running (Colvin and Sawyer, 1969; Wade and Zucker, 1970b). Progesterone seems relatively unimportant to the average amount of wheel running except under conditions when it can inhibit the action of estrogen or substitute for corticosteroids and promote more normal metabolic function as in adrenalectomized animals. Whether or not sex differences in running wheel activity are organized by steroids during the early postnatal period is uncertain. For example, large doses of testosterone propionate (500 to 1250 μg) within 5 days of birth reduce the response of females to activating doses of estrogen given later in life, but eventually the animals exhibit normal activity if treatment is prolonged (see Gerall, 1967; Stern and Janowiak, 1973; Gentry and Wade, 1976b). Prenatal or pre- plus post-natal treatments with androgens have not been studied.

Open-Field Activity

Beginning at about 50 days of age, female rats ambulate more and defecate less than males during open-field tests. Because of the long tradition in animal psychology of interpreting high defecation and low activity as indicative of high "emotionality," it has been assumed by some that female rats are less emotional than males, an assertion that has been disputed by others (see Gray, 1971, vs. Archer, 1975, for both sides of a seemingly endless debate). In contrast to wheel running, where activational effects of estrogen mainly determine activity level, in the open field activational influences of gonadal hormones on active motor behaviors (ambulation and rearing) are rather modest (Quadagno et al., 1972; Bronstein and Hirsch, 1974; Bengelloun et al., 1976; Slater and Blizard, 1976).

Castration at 30 days or later generally does not affect open-field behavior of males, but neonatal castration, especially if combined with prenatal exposure to cyproterone acetate, elevates activity to levels that approximate those seen in females (Scouten et al., 1975; Bengelloun et al., 1976). These observations suggest that exposure to androgens during the perinatal period reduces active open-field behaviors; this has also been demonstrated by studies in which female rats were injected with TP neonatally (Gray et al., 1965; Pfaff and Zigmond, 1971; Blizard and Denef, 1973; Blizard et al., 1975).

Aggression

There are marked species differences in the effects of gonadal hormones on aggression and differences in the testing procedures typically used with each species. Adult male mice are very aggressive toward one another until they establish social dominance relations. Females rarely fight when similarly tested. Hence, the introduction of strangers is an effective technique for inducing aggression in males, especially if the animals have been socially isolated for some time. Both activational and organizational effects of gonadal steroids control aggression in mice. Castration in adulthood abolishes aggressive behavior, and hormone replacement with androgens restores fighting in a dose-dependent fashion (Beeman, 1947; Edwards, 1969). Among androgens, testosterone and androstenedione are most effective in eliciting aggression in castrated males (Erpino and Chappelle, 1973; Luttge and Hall, 1973a), but even "strong" androgens do not elicit much aggression in similarly tested females. Aggression against a male intruder can be increased by injecting females neonatally with testosterone or estrogen (e.g., Bronson and Desjardins, 1968, 1970; Edwards, 1968, 1969; Whitsett et al., 1972).

As would be expected, neonatal castration reduces this kind of aggressiveness in male mice even if given testosterone in adulthood (Edwards, 1969). Again, the effect is time-dependent; castration at 1 day of age is more effective than castration on day 6 or later (Edwards, 1969; Peters et al., 1972). While these findings imply some sort of critical period for the organizing action of testosterone or one of its metabolites, the temporal boundaries of the critical period, if any such thing exists, are not rigidly fixed. Prolonged (20 days long) treatment with TP beginning at day 30 elevates aggression to male levels in female mice given TP injections at testing (Edwards, 1970). One mechanism by which androgens alter aggressiveness is to alter the production of urinary pheromones that stimulate attack in the mouse (e.g., Lee and Griffo, 1973).

In laboratory rats aggression is usually induced by placing pairs of animals in a small chamber and electrifying the grid with a brief but fairly intense shock. Both sexes exhibit considerable "aggression" under these conditions, but males usually fight somewhat more than females, although the sex difference is not large. Castration reduces shock-elicited fighting in males, but the effect takes more than 3 weeks to develop (Hutchinson et al., 1965; Bernard and Paolino, 1975). Organizational effects are also present; neonatal TP in females increases aggression (Powell et al., 1971). Neonatal castration reduces such aggression in males even when they are given TP injections later in life (Conner et al., 1969). The relationship, if any, between such shock-induced aggression and more "natural" social aggressive responses is unknown.

Unlike rats and mice, female *hamsters* exhibit more aggression than males, at least in periods of diestrus. Gonadectomy reduces aggression in both males and females (Payne and Swanson, 1971a,b, 1972a). Combined treatment with estradiol and progesterone completely suppresses fighting in ovariectomized-adrenalectomized females, but neither hormone is very effective alone (Floody and Pfaff, 1977). In castrated males aggression can be increased toward intact males by ovarian transplants and TP or EB injections and toward intact females by progesterone (Payne and Swanson, 1971a, 1972b). Very little is known about organizational effects of gonadal hormones on hamster aggression.

Somewhat surprisingly, neonatal testosterone treatment *increases* aggression in males to levels well above those seen in untreated males (Payne and Swanson, 1972c).

Experiments on hormonal control of aggression in male gerbils have produced highly variable results; both increases and decreases in aggression have been reported after castration or TP injections (see Sayler, 1970; Anisko et al., 1973; Christenson et al., 1973; Lumia et al., 1975; Yahr et al., 1977). Some sort of androgen-dependent, aggression-arousing pheromone also exists in this species (Yahr et al., 1977), but the confusing resulting pattern suggests that variables other than hormonal state must be important. One such factor appears to be the familiarity and neutrality of the testing arena. Gerbils also exhibit sexually dimorphic territorial marking, especially in males (Turner, 1975; Thiessen and Rice, 1976). Testosterone injections increase marking in both males and females, and the magnitude of the increase is much greater in males (Turner, 1975; Thiessen and Rice, 1976). This activational influence of testosterone reflects, in part, a direct action on the brain (Thiessen and Yahr, 1970) and, in part, peripheral changes in the ventral scent glands. Androgens also exert important organizational effects on territorial marking. Neonatal androgen treatment increases responsiveness to subsequent androgen treatment in female gerbils in an age-dependent fashion, while early castration reduces responsiveness to androgen treatment in males in an age-dependent manner (Turner, 1975).

Taste Preferences

Female rats of several strains exhibit a greater preference than males for nutritive (glucose) and nonnutritive (saccharin) solutions (Valenstein et al., 1967; Wade and Zucker, 1969). It is important to realize that ovarian hormones are important mainly for the establishment of saccharin preference, and, once developed, the preference persists following ovariectomy. Ovariectomy greatly reduces acquisition of preference for saccharin, and only combined treatment with estrogen and progesterone restores this ability (Zucker, 1969). Activational effects of testicular hormones are relatively unimportant. Neonatal TP (but not EB) treatment, greatly reduces saccharin preference in females (Wade and Zucker, 1969). Further, feminine saccharin preferences are displayed by male pseudohermaphrodites of the Stanley-Gumbreck strain (Shapiro and Goldman, 1973); these animals are androgen-insensitive because of a genetic defect. In general, gonadal hormones affect saccharin preference in hamsters in much the same way that they do in rats (Zucker et al., 1972).

Female rats also exhibit a greater preference for salt solutions than males (Krecek et al., 1972). This difference is abolished by TP injections in 2-day-old females, but similar injections at 12 days of age are ineffective (Krecek, 1973).

Reactivity to Shock

Female rats are more responsive to electric shock than males, as reflected in lower response thresholds (Paré, 1969; Beatty and Beatty, 1970; Marks and Hobbs, 1972) and shorter escape latencies (Beatty and Beatty, 1970; Davis et al., 1976). There is disagreement regarding the activational role of gonadal hormones in both sexes (see Beatty and Beatty, 1970; Marks and Hobbs, 1972; Marks et al., 1972; Davis et al., 1976; Beatty and Fessler, 1977a). Castration at 50 days of age lowered flinch and shuffle thresholds but left the jump threshold unaltered, while neonatal castration lowered all three of the above shock threshold measures to levels observed in females. Testosterone injections raised shock thresholds of neonatally castrated males to levels of normal males (Beatty and Fessler, 1977a); but Beatty is reluctant to interpret the effects of neonatal castration as evidence for an organizational influence of androgens because neonatal castration ostensibly renders the animal *more* sensitive to TP injections later in life.

Feeding and Body Weight Regulation

As in many mammals, including man, the male rat eats more and weighs more than the female. A slight sex difference in body weight is apparent at birth (Slob and van der Werff ten Bosch, 1975). During the next 4 to 7 weeks of life, males generally remain somewhat heavier than females, but the difference is very small and usually does not attain statistical significance. Beginning about 40 to 50 days of age, a marked divergence in body weight begins and increases throughout life. Hormonal influences contribute to sex differences in body weight in at least three ways:

1. Ovarian hormones, specially estrogen, act to control feeding and body weight by reducing intake as long as body weight exceeds a certain "set point." Progesterone is not important to feeding and body

weight regulation in females with intact adrenals, except that it may inhibit the effects of estrogen (see Wade, 1976). The onset of estrogenic regulation during ontogeny is mainly related to attainment of a minimum body weight level (Zucker, 1972). Actually what is evidently more important is the accumulation of a minimum amount of body fat (Wade, 1976). In the adult female rat, both feeding and food-motivated behavior vary with the estrous cycle; eating and weight are lowest when estrogen titers are high. In ovariectomized animals cyclic patterns of feeding can be induced with intermittent estrogen treatment (Tarttelin and Gorski, 1973). One neural target for estrogen actions on feeding is clearly the ventromedial hypothalamus (VMH). Implants of crystalline estradiol inhibit feeding in gonadectomized rats of both sexes, and estrogen implants in other parts of the hypothalamus do not suppress feeding (e.g., Wade and Zucker, 1970b). However, it is clear that estrogenic suppression of feeding and weight gain involves more than a direct effect on the VMH, since animals with VMH lesions respond to ovariecttomy and estrogen injections in a way that is either nearly normal (King and Cox, 1973; Kemnitz et al., 1977) or attenuated (Beatty et al., 1975b; Nance, 1976), depending on the experimental conditions.

2. Androgens also exert activational effects on feeding and body weight gain. Castration of adult males reduces growth almost immediately and, after some delay, feeding as well. The depression of feeding is persistent, in contrast to the temporary hyperphagia following ovariectomy in the female; body weight gain is also chronically reduced. Replacement with TP increases eating and weight gain in a dose-dependent fashion; moderate doses (below 1 mg/day) stimulate feeding and weight gain. Larger doses actually depress feeding and weight gain below the level of oil-treated castrates. This effect evidently results from aromatization of testosterone to estrogen and can be antagonized by concurrent treatment with progesterone, which by itself has no effect on weight gain in the castrated male. Dihydrotestosterone has only a weak stimullating action on feeding and weight gain (Gentry and Wade, 1976a).

3. Gonadal hormones present during the perinatal period also exert important effects on the level at which body weight will ultimately be regulated. Hormone manipulations during prenatal life often reduce body weight markedly, but these changes are not easy to interpret because of the possibility of nonspecific debilitating effects. The likelihood of this possibility is enhanced because higher than normal mortality rates usually occur after such treatment. Beatty thinks this is the

most reasonable interpretation of the rather frequent observation that prenatal TP treatment *depresses* body weight (e.g., Ward, 1969; Slob and van der Werff ten Bosch, 1975). Moreover, there is little or no difference in body weight between male and female rats castrated at birth; so the role of androgens in the prenatal period is probably not large. However, a single injection of TP or EB shortly after birth increases body weight levels of females in an irreversible fashion. The effect is greater in magnitude if the injections are given to gonadally intact animals, but some difference is observed in ovariectomized females, at least for TP injections (Bell and Zucker, 1971). The effectiveness of early postnatal hormonal treatment in chronically elevating the level at which body weight will be regulated is limited to a tightly demarcated period in postnatal life (Tarttelin et al., 1975), and even treatment for 20 days with large doses (2 mg/day) of TP has no effect on weight regulation when given to prepubertal females (Beatty, 1973b).

Relatively little information regarding the comparative aspects of hormonal control of feeding and body weight in rodents, other than in the rat, is available. In general, the basic effects of hormones on weight regulation seem to be similar in guinea pigs and rats, correcting for differences in the gestation period (Slob et al., 1973; Czaja and Goy, 1975), but the situation is much different in hamsters and gerbils. In the hamster gonadectomy affects neither food intake nor body weight in either sex. Progesterone elevates both measures in castrates of both sexes; testosterone depresses feeding and weight in males but not in females; while estrogen is ineffective in both sexes (Zucker et al., 1972). In the gerbil estrogen and antiestrogens (which are estrogenic in their effects on feeding (Roy and Wade, 1976)) stimulate food intake and weight gain (Roy et al., 1977).

Learning and Performance

Perhaps because of the early discovery of estrus-linked changes in activity, there has been a long-standing tradition in animal (i.e., rodent) psychology to conduct experiments on male rats. According to Beatty, the typical justification for this widely practiced research strategy is to avoid introducing unwanted and extraneous variability that might obscure the phenomena of interest. While this sounds reasonable enough, the strategy has been extremely costly for at least three reasons: (1) We do not possess a very clear idea of the pattern of sex differences in the many tasks that have been studied in laboratory animals over the years. (2) The hoped for reduction in variance between subjects has often not been achieved. (3) The generality of the results of animal learning experiments may be less than is typically assumed.

Despite the long tradition of designing experiments in a manner that precludes discovery of sex differences in behavior, differences in several behaviors have been described. One behavior that has been frequently studied is active avoidance, which is typically studied in one of three test situations: (1) *One way,* where one of two compartments in the apparatus is always safe and the other is potentially dangerous. (2) *Two way (shuttle),* where both sides of a two-compartment chamber are potentially dangerous. (3) *Free operant (Sidman),* in which shock is not signalled by a distinct external stimulus but, instead, is programmed to occur briefly every few seconds.

Female rats generally outperform males during acquisition of each of these tasks. The difference is small and rather undependable in the one-way task, probably because male rats acquire one-way avoidance quite rapidly and there really is not much room for improvement. Sidman avoidance has not been studied extensively, but a sex difference has been reported (Barrett and Ray, 1970). Most of the work on sex differences in acquisition has employed the two-way task.

In rat studies in Beatty's laboratory, organizational influences of androgens during the *prenatal* period were shown to be principally responsible for the sex difference in two-way avoidance acquisition. Activational influences of gonadal hormones seem quite unimportant, since gonadectomy has no effect on performance by either sex (Beatty and Beatty, 1970; Scouten et al., 1975). Although neonatal castration of males did not influence performance, acquisition was improved to the typically female level by combining neonatal gonadectomy with prenatal exposure to the antiandrogen, cyproterone acetate (Scouten et al., 1975). This treatment also feminized their open-field behavior (see above). While these data suggest that organizational effects of androgens on avoidance normally occur prenatally in the rat, other data demonstrate that testosterone can affect performance if given later in development. A single injection of TP at 3 days of age combined with ovariectomy and TP in adulthood caused marked impairment in the performance of females, although neither treatment alone affected avoidance behavior (Beatty and Beatty, 1970). Further, a series of postnatal testosterone injections beginning at birth and ending at 75 days of age tended to depress ($P = 0.06$) acquisition by females in the tests given 2 months after injections ended (Scouten, 1972). There is an interesting parallel between the role of gonadal hormones in this sex-typical behavior and their role in sex differences in learning that is sensitive to orbital-frontal lesions in rhesus monkeys (see below).

Female rats (Denti and Epstein, 1972; Beatty et al., 1973; Bengelloun et al., 1976) and gerbils (Riddell et al., 1975) exhibit inferior performance in tests of passive avoidance behavior. As yet, no influence of gonadal hormones has been demonstrated, since castration at various ages from birth to adulthood does not affect performance in rats (Bengelloun et al., 1976).

Adult female rats acquire efficient performance on a differential reinforcement of low rates of response (DRL) schedule more rapidly than males (Beatty, 1973a; Kearly et al., 1974). At first, it appeared that activational effects of ovarian hormones were mainly responsible for the sex difference, since ovariectomy greatly impaired performance (Beatty, 1973a). However, two attempts to replicate this result have failed; so the role of ovarian hormones in this sexual dimorphism is not established (Lentz et al., 1978).* Similarly, there is no evidence that androgens contribute to the sex difference in DRL acquisition, since neither adult nor neonatal castration alters the performance of males (Beatty, 1973a; Beatty et al., 1975a). The possible influence of gonadal hormones during the prenatal period has not yet been examined.

With a few exceptions (e.g., Corey, 1930), studies that have observed sex differences in *maze learning* in rats have found that males are superior (e.g., Tryon, 1931; McNemar and Stone, 1932; Barrett and Ray, 1970; Krasnoff and Weston, 1976). The tasks that are most sensitive to the sex difference are complex mazes (e.g., the Lashley III maze) with many blind alleys. Such an apparatus is really an open field with many additional walls, and, consequently, it is not surprising that females make more errors since their greater level of activity and exploratory behavior translates rather directly into "errors" in the maze. Beatty is not aware of any systematic attempt to examine activational effects of gonadal hormones; but, if these complex mazes are really just elaborate open fields, only modest effects would be expected. Organizational effects of androgens would be anticipated, and there is one confirming report.

*C.M. Bierley and W.W. Beatty, unpublished data.

Stewart and colleagues (1975) reported that neonatal TP injections improved the performance of females in the Lashley III maze almost to the level of normal male controls. The same treatment also masculinized open-field behavior. There is also a report of a failure of prenatal or neonatal TP to affect Lashley III maze performance of females (Machado-Magalhaes and de Araujo-Carlini, 1974), but those workers also failed to observe a difference in Lashley III maze performance between normal males and females. A recent experiment by Beckwith and colleagues (1977) reported a sex difference in the acquisition and reversal of a black-white discrimination in a Thompson-Bryant box. Males required fewer trials to criterion during both acquisition and reversal, and only performance of males improved as a result of neonatal treatment with melanocyte-stimulating hormone.

Recently, Chambers (1976) reported that male rats extinguish a *conditioned taste aversion* more slowly than females. Gonadectomy reduced the persistence of the aversion in males but did not affect performance by females. Testosterone treatment increased the resistance to extinction of females and castrated males. While it is possible that the phenomenon described by Chambers is a special case of altered taste preference or of extinction of passive avoidance behavior, the nature of the effects of hormonal manipulations in adulthood on taste aversion is different from the effects of similar manipulations on taste preferences or passive avoidance (cf. Zucker, 1969; Bengelloun et al., 1976). Beatty is not aware of any data on the effects of perinatal hormone manipulations on taste aversions.

Sex Differences in Response to Brain Damage

Goldman and colleagues (1974) reported that the effects of orbital-frontal lesions in rhesus monkeys were both sex- and age-dependent. Using three tests (object reversal, delayed response, and delayed alternation), they observed deficits in males but not in females if brain damage and testing occurred before 15 to 18 months of age. If the operations and tests occurred later in life, impairments were observed in both sexes. Since the publication of that paper, Goldman and colleagues have done additional work that demonstrates the following: (1) In young monkeys (75 days old) males perform better than females on the object reversal task, but this difference disappears as development progresses. (2) A series of postnatal TP injections (birth to 46 days of age) or prenatal TP treatment improves performance of females to about the level of young males. The number of animals in the prenatal TP group is small, but it is clear that they are not better than the postnatal despite more extensive somatic virilization. (3) Early castration does not affect male performance. The implication of these results is that androgens may affect the rate of maturation of portions of the brain that are involved in competence in performing object reversal problems but which are probably not primarily steroid targets. It will be interesting to see what happens to the performance of males exposed to antiandrogens prenatally and castrated at birth. If their performance on object reversal at 75 days is reduced, the interpretation advanced by Goldman and colleagues would be nicely supported. In addition, there is an obvious parallel between the type of hormonal control that seems to be involved in this dimorphic behavior in the monkey and what Beatty has observed in active avoidance behavior in rats (see below).

The effects of septal lesions on emotionality in the rat are now known to be sex-, age-, and hormone-dependent. Lesions at 7 days of age and after 55 days of age result in full appearance of hyperemotionality, but similar lesions at 25 days of age are ineffective and at 30 or 45 days of age "hyperemotionality" is quite transient (Johnson, 1972; Phillips and Lieblich, 1972). Gonadectomy in males at any time other than between ages 23 to 30 days has no effect on the development of hyperemotionality when lesions are made in adulthood; between 23 to 30 days (especially 26 to 29 days of age) gonadectomy greatly attenuates the hyperemotionality from adult septal lesions (Phillips and Lieblich, 1972; Lieblich et al., 1974; Bengelloun et al., 1976). Female rats that normally show hyperemotionality even if lesions are made when they are weanlings do not show hyperemotionality if lesioned at 25 days of age if they have been given neonatal TP treatment. Conversely, neonatally castrated males show hyperemotionality from septal destruction at 25 days of age, when normal males do not exhibit the septal rage syndrome (Phillips and Deol, 1973). These results imply a complex age-dependent action of androgens in which neonatal exposure to androgen triggers some mechanism that reduces the organism's emotional reactivity following the lesion. Evidently, subsequent exposure to androgens during a remarkably tightly bounded period before puberty reverses this process, whatever it may be. The effects of septal lesions on open field, active avoidance, and passive avoidance behavior do not seem to depend on gonadal hormones, at least not in the same way as emotionality (Bengelloun et al., 1976). Unfortunately, sex differences in the effects of septal lesions on consummatory and operant behavior (Kondo and Lorens, 1971; Lorens and Kondo, 1971) have not been analyzed with regard to their dependence on gonadal hormones.

Lenard and colleagues (1975) reported that large lesions of the globus pallidus had different effects on the duration of aphagia and adipsia in male and female rats. Despite intragastric feedings, most males died without recovering voluntary feeding or drinking, but most females survived and recovered ingestive behaviors. Exactly the same pattern of sex differences in feeding occurred after intrapallidal injection of the neurotoxin, 6-hydroxydopamine (Lenard, 1977). Using smaller lesions of the pallidus, which did not cause aphagia or adipsia in either sex or affect open-field behavior, Beatty and Siders (1977) observed impaired acquisition of two-way avoidance in both sexes, but one-way avoidance acquisition was retarded by the lesions only in males. In a parallel series of studies Studelska and Beatty (1978) observed sex-dependent effects of lesions in the ventral part of the caudate. These lesions caused transient aphagia and adipsia of comparable duration in both sexes, but impaired two-way avoidance behavior only in males. Open-field behavior and acquisition of one-way avoidance behavior were not impaired in either sex. They have also examined the influence of gonadectomy in adulthood on the effects of the ventral caudate lesions. Castration abolished the deficit in avoidance that was observed after lesions in gonadally intact males, but ovariectomy had no influence on performance in females regardless of whether or not they also had lesions. Treatment of male castrates with TP, EB, or dihydrotestosterone propionate seems to restore the effectiveness of the lesion in males, but TP injections do not produce impairments in females with ventral caudate lesions. To date, Beatty's experiments with injections of antiestrogen (MER-25 or CI 628) or an antiandrogen (cyproterone acetate) in gonadally intact males with ventral caudate lesions have not revealed any effect of these antagonists on avoidance behavior, possibly because the antiestrogens mimic the effect of EB.

The effects of both ventromedial hypothalamic and lateral hypothalamic lesions on feeding behavior and body weight regulation indicate sex differences. When the VMH is damaged by electrolytic lesions, gold thioglucose injections, or by knife cuts lateral to the VMH region, hyperphagia and obesity are more frequently observed (or these effects are greater in magnitude) in females than in males (Valenstein et al., 1969; Wright and Turner, 1973; see also Wade, 1976; Kemnitz et al., 1977). Wade (1976) has suggested that the effect of the VMH lesion is to abolish the sex difference in food intake and in body weight gain that exists in neurologically intact males and females; i.e., after VMH damage males and females eat and gain weight at comparable rates. However, in a few studies (e.g., Valenstein et al., 1969) females gained absolutely more weight than males after VMH lesions.

Following LH lesions there is a sex difference in the level at which body weight is ultimately regulated. Both males and females exhibit aphagia and adipsia after lateral hypothalamic lesions, followed by partial recovery of ingestive behavior; but males, more reliably than females, regulate body weight at chronically lower than normal levels (Powley and Keesey, 1970). Female rats with lateral hypothalamic lesions can regulate body weight at more nearly normal levels (Harrell and Balagura, 1975; see also Wade, 1976). These sex differences in response to hypothalamic injury are consistent with a model of sex differences in feeding recently proposed by Nance and Gorski (1975). These authors note that sex differences between neurologically intact males and females on measures such as preference for strong saccharine solutions and diurnal rhythms in meal taking are qualitatively similar to the changes in feeding caused by VMH or lateral hypothalamic lesions, respectively. Thus, the feeding behavior of a normal male resembles that of an animal with a VMH lesion, while the normal female's feeding behavior is more like that of an animal with a lateral hypothalamic lesion. According to the model, neural systems that control feeding are intrinsically biased to develop in the feminine direction with an active VMH that restrains feeding and weight gain (possibly in response to changing estrogen levels; see above). Perinatal exposure to androgens might modify the development of the VMH to weaken its inhibitory control over feeding, a plausible possibility, since the VMH has been implicated as a target area for the organizational actions of androgens on neuroendocrine control mechanisms (Nadler, 1973). Moreover, neonatal treatment of female rats with TP reduces the effects of adult VMH lesions on feeding (Valenstein, 1968) and masculinizes taste preferences (e.g., Nance, 1976). However, it is not clear from the model why castration in adulthood should enhance the effectiveness of VMH lesions on feeding and weight gain in males (Kemnitz et al., 1977).

Clearly, additional work is necessary to evaluate the interactions of gonadal hormones and brain lesions that affect feeding and other behaviors. This work is needed to resolve discrepancies that have already appeared, but it is likely to be especially fruitful for another reason: brain monoamine systems that are affected by many of the lesions described above are known to be involved in many aspects of sexual and nonreproductive behavior. Recent work has shown that there are sex differences in monoamine levels in many brain regions that are influenced by organizational and activational effects of gonadal hormones (Vaccari et al., 1977; Crowley et al., 1978).

Sexually Dimorphic Behavior in Birds

In an "ideal" bird the release of FSH by the pituitary is influenced by day length. In males FSH leads to testosterone secretion by the testes; in females, to estrogen secretion by the ovary. The presence of high levels of testosterone in males leads to male courtship. Male courtship, in turn, further stimulates FSH secretion in females so that still more estrogen is produced. Estrogen in females induces nest building, which is followed by progesterone release, leading to ovulation, incubation, and parental behavior. However, there are 8,580 living species of birds, and birds as a group show gross variability in their sexual behavior. The ideal bird is a rather elusive creature. Some specific examples of the above-mentioned interactions between hormones, environmental factors, and avian sexual behavior are to be found in Witschi (1961), Lofts and Murton (1973), Lehrman (1964), Hinde (1970, pp. 633-640), and Hutchison (1975).

According to Nottebohm, sexually dimorphic behavior in birds falls into two rough categories that show considerable overlap: spacing behavior, which is particularly well developed in males, and reproductive behavior. When reproduction calls for spacing, the same behavior may be used to repel other males and attract females.

Spacing behaviors have the effect of apportioning resources between members of a population. The resource in question may be space or food, as when a bird stakes out a territory that includes potential nest sites as well as food resources adequate to feed itself, its mate, and its progeny. Advertising the ownership of such a large territory is usually entrusted to vocal displays, such as songs, which carry over considerable distance and penetrate dense cover. This type of breeding territory and territorial defense is common to many songbirds (Howard, 1920). In some cases spacing efforts are restricted to claiming a nest site and a minimum amount of space surrounding it. This behavior is typical of colonial breeders, such as many seabirds (Tinbergen, 1953; Nelson, 1965) or some of the weaver finches (Collias and Collias, 1967). Spacing efforts may also focus on a display arena. In this case males can be very close to each other, but defend exclusive rights to the few square or cubic yards where they advertise their reproductive availability. Display arenas have been described for grouse (Hjorth, 1970; Wiley, 1973, 1974), ruff (Hogan-Warburg, 1966), manakins (Lill, 1974, 1976), and some hummingbirds (Snow, 1968; Wiley, 1971).

Territorial displays that lead to these different types of spacing are species typical and often stereotyped, what ethologists call "fixed-action patterns" (see review in Hinde, 1970; Marler and Hamilton, 1966; Barlow, 1977). With the exception of song in some groups of birds, the motor programs responsible for the fixed-action pattern are thought to be under genetic control. The cooing behavior of doves is a good example of a fixed-action pattern used in both spacing and courtship. Cooing develops normally in young squabs reared by foster species (Lade and Thorpe, 1964) or deafened soon after hatching (Nottebohm and Nottebohm, 1971). Thus, the stereotypy and species-typical characters of these vocalizations are not learned by imitation or by reference to auditory feedback. Hybrid doves produce cooing patterns that often bear no resemblance to the rhythmic patterns of either parental species, and in extreme cases the cooing of the hybrid is "completely disorganized" (Lade and Thorpe, 1964).

Genes may always control some parameters of sexually dimorphic avian vocal repertoires, but in some groups this control is sufficiently lax to allow for considerable amounts of learning. The song of oscine songbirds and that of some hummingbirds fall into this category, as does the vocal repertoire of parrots and their relatives (for review, see Nottebohm, 1972). In all these cases, as the bird develops its vocal repertoire, it modifies vocal output until the auditory feedback it generates matches an auditory expectation. This matching process is interrupted by deafening (Konishi, 1965; Nottebohm, 1968; review by Konishi and Nottebohm, 1969). The vocal patterns are usually so improbable or complex that it is fair to assume that for any one individual they constitute novel motor programs that would not have occurred in the absence of vocal learning.

Singing behavior is better developed among male than among female songbirds, though females of many species sing. For example, the hen of the European robin sings freely in the autumn, when male and female robins defend individual territories (Lack, 1943). Many other examples could be presented (Nottebohm, 1975), though as a group they confirm the view that, even in species where females sing, under normal conditions the incidence of such song is far below that of males. Exceptions to this are cases where both members of a pair engage in singing duets (for review, see Armstrong, 1963; Thorpe and North, 1965). It seems possible that, even in species where female song has been judged to be a rare event, it serves a purpose. For example, bow-cooing is a typical male behavior of aggressive or courting ring doves. Its occurrence is controlled by hypothalamic centers and requires testosterone (Hutchison, 1967, 1975). Yet both male and female ring doves bow-coo until they are 3 to 4 months old. Bow-cooing disappears from the female repertoire as the birds develop into breeding condition, which occurs at 5 to 6 months (Nottebohm and Nottebohm, 1971). Whether bow-cooing in young female ring doves is a meaningful reflection of the developing endocrine system or an important step for normal socialization is not known.

We can assume that female oscine songbirds, which normally sing, develop their song as a vocal learning process, as the males do. An intriguing example is the sexually dimorphic vocal repertoire of the Indian hill mynah. In this species males in a particular area imitate calls of other males in that area, whereas females imitate only female calls (Bertram, 1970). Such sex-restricted imitation depends on recognition of the sex of the potential model, not a simple task in a species lacking morphological sexual dimorphism. In some species, such as the South American rufous-collared sparrow, female song may occur rarely and then only early in the breeding season. Nottebohm pointed out that two female sparrows that he has collected produced songs that were close replicas of the dialect characteristic of the local population. The dialect is known to be a learned trait for the local population; therefore, by inference, the two females had also learned it.

Nest building is another complex sexually dimorphic trait. The extent of male or female participation varies among species. Both sexes of ring doves cooperate in nest construction, the male usually gathering material and carrying it to the female, who stands at the nest site and constructs the nest (Lehrman, 1964). It is the female canary that constructs the nest (e.g., Hinde and Steel, 1966), but the male European wren constructs a number of nests. After the male forms a pair bond with a female, she will select one of the nests and provide the soft lining (Armstrong, 1955). Multiple nest building is also shown by male long-billed marsh wrens (Verner and Engelsen, 1970) and by male weaver-birds. This latter African finch weaves a domed nest out of grass or palm leaf strips (Collias and Collias, 1962), and the quality of the nest improves with practice (Collias and Collias, 1973).

Song learning and nest building are both under hormonal control and experience can play a role in both. However, they may differ in that song learning leads to the acquisition of new motor patterns, whereas improvements in nest building may result merely from better selection and handling of building materials.

There is at least one case where the genetic contribution to nest building has been demonstrated. Some African lovebirds of the genus *Agapornis* carry nesting material in their beak. Other lovebirds of the same genus, but different species, carry nesting material by sticking it under the feathers of their rump. Although hybrids try both patterns of carrying nesting material, they never succeed in rump transportation. With practice these more ineffectual attempts are abandoned (Dilger, 1962).

Vocal displays and nest building were emphasized above because they are sexually dimorphic behaviors particularly well developed in birds; but other sexual behaviors are still to be considered. With the exception of copulation and egg laying, the performer's sex in other reproductive roles varies considerably among species and groups of birds. In this sense birds show a remarkable diversity of evolutionary adaptations. For example, something as basic as incubation can be the sole responsibility of females, as in the case of fowl, ducks, hummingbirds, manakins, and most oscine songbirds where the female has a dull coloration. In doves and some parrots both sexes incubate, though the female still does more and is responsible for the longer night shift. In some shorebirds the decision of who incubates what can be a complicated one: in the spotted sandpiper, males incubate the first clutches and polyandrous females share in the incubation of the final clutch (Hays, 1972). In the sanderling, two clutches are laid in separate nests and the pair bond dissolves before incubation begins. Each member of the pair incubates one of the clutches and attends the ensuing young (Parmelee, 1970; Parmelee and Payne, 1973). In some groups of birds females have liberated themselves of all maternal chores other than egg laying: in rheas, tinamous, jacanas (Jenni and Collier, 1972), and phalaropes (Höhn, 1967), it is the male that does all the incubating. Interestingly, in species such as domestic fowl, mallard, and red-winged blackbird, where the female has retained sole responsibility for incubation and care of the young, there is a higher content of testosterone in the testis than in the ovaries; in pigeons, where both sexes share in incubation and care of the young, and in the phalarope, where these roles are the sole responsibility of males, testosterone content (in micrograms per gram of tissue) is higher in the ovaries than in the testis (Höhn and Cheng, 1967). Interpretation of this suggested relationship is difficult, since the relation between ovarian testosterone content and follicular events has not been worked out. The higher ovarian than testicular concentration of testosterone may be a transitory and not a persisting characteristic.

In some truly modern species, neither sex builds a nest nor incubates. These are the brood parasites, such as the New World's cowbirds (genus *Molothrus* (Rothstein, 1975; Friedmann et al., 1977)), Africa's parasitic indigo birds (genus *Vidua* (Nicolai, 1964; Payne, 1973)), and the South American black-headed duck (Weller, 1967). But perhaps the most remarkable arrangement of all is that found among the megapodes of the South Pacific. In this group of galliformes, incubation heat is solely provided by environmental sources. Brush turkeys, for example, construct mounds of plant material and the male regularly tests the temperature of the mound by probing with its bill. In the first burst of fermentation, the temperature of mounds rises to a high level and the male digs into the top, turning and mixing the material. Not until the temperature is declining does he permit the female to approach and lay eggs. Throughout the incubation period the male remains in charge of the mound and exercises some control over its temperature (Frith, 1964).

Nest building, copulation, incubation, and parental duties are usually preceded by courtship. Evolutionary forces have used every possible stratagem to create the most varied courtship patterns. Australian bowerbirds have evolved polvchrome nuptial palaces decorated with flowers, berries, and shells (Gilliard, 1969). The Australian lyrebird has evolved a baroque and exquisite song dance. Such hypertrophied male displays seem to occur in species with very brief sexual encounters. While the males are polygamous, all postcopulatory reproductive roles are left to the females. In the more common situation of monogamous species cementing the bond between the sexes, all steps leading to copulation are slower and require some degree of intimacy. Well-worked examples are the displays of grebes (Huxley, 1914), gulls (Tinbergen, 1953), ducks (Lorenz, 1941), and some songbirds (e.g., Marler, 1956). Many of these behaviors are ritualized (e.g., Morris, 1957) and lend themselves well as visual signals conveying the reproductive intentions of both partners.

Courtship displays convey sexual and species-specific information. Their most obvious role is to ensure that sexual interactions occur between members of the same species and opposite sex. Courtship is also thought to *synchronize* the behavioral rhythms of prospective partners, *trigger* adequate behavioral responses, and *direct* these responses so that the interacting individuals are properly oriented (Tinbergen, 1951; Lehrman, 1964).

Courtship displays often include two or three interacting motivations, subsumed as aggression, fear, and sexual drive (Tinbergen, 1952, 1954; Hinde, 1953; Moynihan, 1955; Morris, 1957). Successive displays are supposed to allay the element of fear, reduce aggression, and permit the full expression of the sexual drive. This theory is supported by the fact that many courtship displays include components or modified parts otherwise known to occur as part of pure threat or pure escape behaviors. The overlap in courtship between sexual and agonistic tendencies is understandable if we think that the close proximity required by copulation necessitates a degree of boldness by the sex initiating the encounter. This boldness, or aggression, is otherwise encountered in dominance relations, for example, in wintering flocks, where aggression secures access to a scarce resource such as food. Those experienced with the displays of doves and domestic fowl must have pondered whether all male courtship has not evolved from these more primitive, highly aggressive approaches. It is interesting that in some primates we see the reverse borrowing of display elements; in this case sexual displays are used in agonistic situations so that, for example, presenting and mounting are, respectively, extreme forms of submissiveness and dominance, and in this context they can be shown by either sex (Wickler, 1967).

The dependence of avian sexual displays on an adequate complement of hormones has been forcefully demonstrated by the work of Lehrman and associates at Rutgers, and by Hinde and collaborators at Cambridge (Lehrman, 1964; Cheng and Lehrman, 1975; Hinde, 1965, 1970, p. 636). The work of these authors has also shown how external stimuli, such as day length, access to nesting material, and occurrence of sexual displays, affect levels of circulating hormones; and how the opportunity to perform certain behaviors, in turn, brings about further hormonal changes. From this viewpoint the courting interactions between members of a pair can be seen as a way of bringing into step the physiology of both partners in preparation for the subsequent parental duties of incubation and care of the young. It should be noted, though, that in birds as in mammals, despite the information content of sexual displays and despite the hormonal control of these displays, "mistakes" can occur, leading to homosexual behavior in male-male and female-female pairs (e.g., Buchanan, 1966; Hunt and Hunt, 1977).

There is one other potential role of sexual displays that has not yet received proper attention: the role as *fitness predictors.* Each sex runs the risk of selecting as a mate an inferior individual. In polygamous species with display arenas, only a few males succeed in attracting females. These successful birds are older ones and hold central territories obtained after months, sometimes years, of fierce competition (Wiley, 1973, 1974; Lill, 1976). Their chance of leaving progeny is maximized by inseminating all comers. Females minimize their risk of choosing an inferior partner by selecting these central "winners." In the more common situation of monogamous species, each individual, regardless of sex, should strive to find an optimal partner. Traits sought after should be endurance to survive environmental extremes; aggressiveness in competing for mates, territories, and food; a physiology honed for optimal food utilization; disease resistance, etc. Each sex should seek a partner that will excel in the fullfillment of parental duties, that will show zeal in incubation and efficiency in feeding and defending its young. Much as in the old times, the father of the bride demanded a financial report from his aspiring son-in-law, the male and female of a prospective pair should demand from each other a fitness report. As courtship displays evolve, each sex should seek in its counterpart behaviors that are good predictors of genetic fitness and future parental performance, and should respond favorably to those behaviors. The influence of nutrition on reproduction has been described in several mammals (Sadleir, 1969). Recent studies suggest that under-nutrition affects the levels of gonadotropic hormone-releasing hormones, which in turn affects testosterone secretion (Millar and Fairall, 1976). In chicken and white-crowned sparrows, restricted access to food results in reduced testicular size (Parker and Arscott, 1964; Miller, 1970), and, presumably, such testis secretes less testosterone. Success at finding food is surely one component of fitness. Behaviors dependent on testosterone levels, such as aggression and birdsong, could give a good quantitative report on this aspect of the fitness of an individual; thus, a female may be well advised in responding selectively to such displays. Nottebohm has less of a feeling for what may be a fitness predictor in females. In the golden-headed manakin females visiting a display arena respond to a courting male by performing some of the acrobatics used by displaying males (Lill, 1976, p. 12). In the chaffinch the female's initial response is submissive, yet becomes more aggressive before copulation (Marler, 1956). In gannets females approach males in a submissive manner and males receive them aggressively, biting them (Nelson, 1965, pp. 266-268). This agonistic nature of the bonding ceremony is so marked that Nelson remarks that male aggression and female tolerance must have evolved in linkage. We may wonder whether male aggression and female tolerance to aggression may not be a measure of the same underlying factor, an element of toughness or "courage." Much as it takes courage to attack, it also takes courage not to turn and flee. Are female displays controlled by a molecule or molecules whose circulating levels, as suggested for male testosterone, bear a relation to long-term health and reproductive fitness? The choice of partner should be equally meticulous by male and female. Male displays tend to be vigorous, boisterous: a surplus of nests, cascades of song, strutting, parading, and aggression. If these are, in part at least, ways of displaying fitness, we can only conclude that females are more subtle in putting forth their case!

Why is it that a particular hormone, or mix of hormones, has come to influence the ontogeny and manifestation of various reproductive displays? Why is it that a particular set of courtship behaviors has become necessary for pair formation and necessary to achieve the synchrony required by sexual reproduction? Part of the answer, at least, may be that each sex demands a credible fitness report from its future partner.

Sexual Dimorphisms in Nonhuman Primates

While perhaps not so numerous as avian species, the 11 families and 60 genera of primates present an astonishing array of adaptations in morphology and behavior. In size alone, they vary from the pygmy marmoset and mouse lemur *(Microcebus),* which average only about 70 g in adult weight, to the huge gorilla, which may attain an adult body weight (in males) of 275 kg. Not less varied are their social adaptations, which range from the virtually semisolitary life-style of the orangutan to those complex, highly structured societies (some containing more than 200 individuals) characteristic of some monkeys and baboons. A number of recent books summarize the social adaptations of nonhuman primates, especially those from the Old World, whose evolutionary biology more closely parallels that of human beings (Southwick, 1963; Kummer, 1971; Rowell, 1972; Lancaster, 1975). These summaries are based on data gathered during field studies, and, accordingly, the results are primarily descriptive and do not represent the level of analysis of causation that normally characterizes experimental work. Similarly, the observations have been carried out by different workers having different viewpoints and interested in different problems. These differences, however, do not in any way account for the recorded differences in social adaptations any more than they are able to account for reported concordances and similarities. Thus, the existence of monogamous pair bonds that may last throughout adult life is an established fact for species as distantly related as the gibbon ape of Asia and some of the marmosets of South America. The occurrence of monogamous mating in these primates is associated with an absence of sexual dimorphism in body size, and, perhaps to a lesser extent, with an absence of sexual dimorphism in behavior (Carpenter, 1942). For the marmoset, even parental care tends to be equally provided by both parents except for the restriction of lactation to the female (Eisenberg, 1972). For nonhuman primates, in general, it can be said that a strong relationship exists between sexual dimorphism in body size and the system of mating that is characteristic of a species (Leutenegger, 1978).

Variations in social adaptations have encouraged field workers to develop a primitive classificatory system delineating the basic social unit for each species. Most often, this basic social unit has two features that differ conspicuously among different populations. They are (1) the socionomic index (the ratio of adult females to adult males), and (2) the system of mating. These two features are independent. Thus, when the socionomic index is 1.00, the system of mating may be monogamy with permanent or enduring pair bonding, and the basic social unit is the bonded pair and their offspring, or it may be complete promiscuity with transient pair bonding during the consortship. Generally among Old World terrestrial monkeys and baboons, the socionomic index is greater than 1.00, sometimes approaching 4.00 in rhesus (Lindburg, 1971); but the system of mating can be either promiscuous or an entirely different sort, such as the harem type.

Although an association clearly exists between habitat and the basic social unit of nonhuman primate groups, this association represents a remote evolutionary causation (i.e., selection for a particular adaptation), and contemporary changes in habitat are often without effect in modifying the species-specific social unit. Kummer (1971), for example, describes specific social organizations for hamadryas and anubis baboons despite overlapping geographic habitats. Hamadryas baboons typically have evolved a three-level society consisting of (1) the troop, (2) the medium-sized band, and (3) the one-male unit, which consists of a single male and his permanently bonded adult females and their dependent offspring. Anubis baboons, in contrast, have evolved a multimale troop consisting of a small group of males living continuously with a large number of females and their dependent offspring. In this latter social organization the mating system is accurately described as promiscuous, and only brief and temporary bonds occur between mating individuals. In the former case (the hamadryas), mating, though polygynous, is restricted to the one-male unit, and matings with females outside this unit have not been reported even for females belonging to the same band or troop. In their natural habitats, anubis and hamadryas also differ in their sleeping habits, the former roosting in trees and the latter lodging on cliffs.

As Kummer (1971) reports, anubis and hamadryas occupy adjacent niches in the Awash National Park in Ethiopia. At the boundary of their niches, hybrids are found that have a curious mixture of hamadryas and anubis characteristics in their social organization. Where there are one-male groups, these are small and unstable, and the successes of males in forming harems are meager. Within this park, the ecological transition from forest to cliff country corresponded exactly with changes in sleeping habits for both species, such that anubis now slept in cliffs and hamadryas in trees, but social organization was not similarly affected by the ecological change. "Anubis groups without one-male groups, hamadryas troops with one-male groups, and the in-between societies of the hybrids all occurred in the same canyon habitat" (Kummer, 1971, p. 135). Thus, while some behavioral traits are clearly flexible and adaptable to changing habitats, others (like social organization) are more rigid and more constantly associated with genotype than with habitat.

The tendency to pair bonding and monogamous mating is so strong among marmosets that it can be manifest even in the laboratory environment when a female is housed simultaneously with two males (Epple, 1972). Similar dispositional tendencies have been noted for the monogamous New World titi monkey (Mason, 1978). Thus, the tendency for the bonded male and female with their dependent offspring to constitute the basic unit may be genetically rather than environmentally determined, and it is conceivable that the multimale troop might be genetically based as well.

Efforts to characterize the structure of nonhuman primate societies at levels more analytic than mere description of the ratio of males to females and the systems of mating involved have relied on two different, but not necessarily mutually exclusive, concepts: (1) the dominance hierarchy and (2) social roles. Within the context of sexually dimorphic behaviors, both concepts have relevance.

Dominance is most often defined in terms of performance measures. The defining behaviors are either the frequency of aggressive behaviors, the frequency of submissive behaviors, or the number of troop members toward which either of these behaviors is displayed. Less often dominance is determined by dyadic competition for a valued incentive. For example, the observer may toss an apple approximately midway between two monkeys and record which obtains possession. Obviously, use of the term dominance should not go beyond its defining operations, but it nearly always does so. To say that animal A is dominant to animal B merely summarizes a behavioral relationship between them, and it neither "explains" nor provides insight into the reasons for that relationship. Nevertheless, many workers use the term dominance as though it explains why animal A aggresses animal B and the reverse never or only rarely occurs. Despite its shortcomings and misuses, most Old World terrestrial monkeys and baboons display hierarchical organization of their aggressive-submissive interactions. One or a few of the animals are never threatened or aggressed by the others, and, at the opposite end of the hierarchy, one or a few animals are threatened or aggressed by nearly everyone on occasions of dyadic interaction that are appropriate to the elicitation of such behaviors. Quite regularly among these species, one or a few males are at the top of this hierarchy. This is a regularity that cannot be accounted for by physical size, since, clearly, if that were the only determinant all adult males in the society would be distributed among the top ranks, and this is not what occurs. For our purposes, however, it is important only to note that the top ranks are consistently associated in some species with the male sex.

In nonhuman primate societies for which dominance hierarchies are inappropriate, or as an alternative to that notion, investigators have developed and utilized the concept of social role. First suggested for rhesus monkeys by Bernstein and Sharpe (1966), the concept has also been useful for the baboon (Rowell, 1966), the African vervet (Gartlan, 1968), and Japanese macaques (Eaton, 1976). Social roles for members of these societies are, in part, related to age and dominance rank, but even more strikingly to sex. Thus, Eaton (1976) describes a role specific to the alpha male Japanese macaque (directing movement of the troop). In addition, subleader males assist the alpha male in "policing" and defending the troop against predators. Adult females, in contrast, do not take part in these activities to any great extent, and their role is described primarily as raising and protecting infants and defending female allies in intra-troop aggressive encounters. For vervet monkeys, Gartlan (1968) describes interfering in intra-group aggressing as exclusively an alpha male role, and the chasing of intruders out of the group territory as a role for the alpha and juvenile males. In his study, females were more often the initiators and receivers of friendly approaches than males of any age class. Gartlan emphasizes that learning plays a significant part in the assumption of social roles. Although biological factors may determine the range of social roles an animal performs, "there is no evidence that particular roles are associated with different [genetically determined] levels of biological fitness . . ." (Gartlan, 1968, p. 115).

It should never be assumed from what has been said that all Old World primate groups are organized in such a way that an alpha male can always be identified, or that the role of the alpha male is the same from one species to another. For example, the *patas* monkey is an Old World terrestrial species generally found in one-male units or groups. But the females in the band lead the movements of the group and the single male does not play the kind of leadership role characteristic of the hamadryas male with his harem (Kummer, 1971). Moreover, females in the *patas* band seem quite able to control which male will remain with the band through the mechanism of initiating copulation only with the preferred male and aggression directed toward the non-preferred male (Gutstein, 1978). Under the social system of the *patas*, the single male in the one-male band may not be the alpha animal at all, and social roles conceptualized as stereotypes of masculinity may be the prerogatives of females (Rowell, 1978).

In general, studies of feral primates have paid less attention to social roles of infants and juveniles than to those of adults. While most workers would agree that primates as a class are unique in their prolongation of the period of extrauterine dependency of offspring, only generalizations concerning its significance have been offered. Thus, Lancaster (1975) points out that the freedom of offspring from the responsibilities of adult social roles provides a protracted opportunity to learn complex social skills essential for later roles. The primary vehicle for learning such skills is postulated to be play, and juveniles of most primate species display high levels of social play. In this context, if the division of adult social roles according to sex that characterizes some primates is considered, it is not too surprising that forms of juvenile play also differ according to sex. Males show rougher and more vigorous forms of play than females, and females show more interest in individuals younger than themselves than males do. The former of these juvenile patterns, namely the disposition of males to show rougher and more vigorous play than females, has been studied in the laboratory as a sexually differentiated trait in rhesus monkeys (Goy and Phoenix, 1971). In that study, males and females taken from their mother at 3 months of age were shown to display differentiated patterns of development of rough-and-tumble play. Males performed this behavior about twenty times more frequently than females. More recently, the development of this behavior has been studied in a situation in which mothers and infants of both sexes were continuously present throughout the first year of life. The presence of mothers throughout this period of development neither diminished nor enhanced the sex difference in performance (Figure 1), and males continued to outperform females.

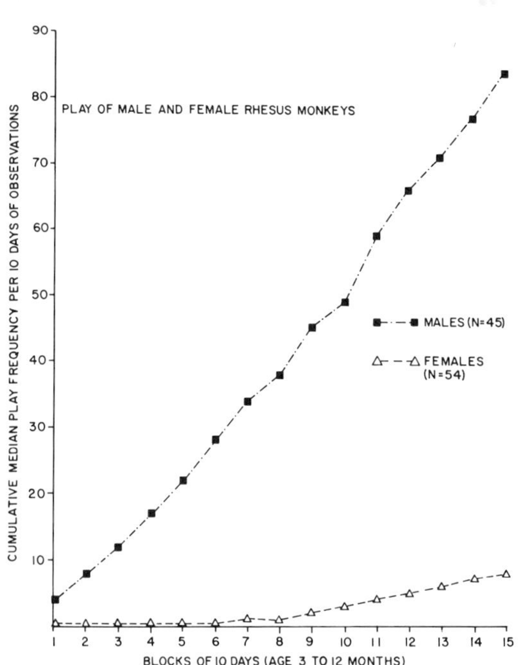

Figure 1. Sex differences in the frequency of performance of rough play by rhesus monkeys during the first year of life. [Goy]

In another study aimed at determining whether the presence of males actively inhibited performance by juvenile females, groups containing only mothers and their female offspring were studied (Goldfoot and Wallen, 1978). The frequencies of performance of rough-and-tumble play by juvenile females reared with only females present were not different from those shown by females reared in heterosexual groups. This finding is in essential agreement with one previously reported (Goy, 1968) that utilized a mother-free testing situation. Thus, the tendency of female rhesus monkeys *not* to engage frequently in rough play is not easily modified by environmental influences.

The tendency of males to display high frequencies of rough play is not related to secretions of the testis after birth. When male rhesus monkeys were castrated at any time from the day of birth to 3 months of age, their subsequent display of rough play equalled that of normal intact males (Figure 2). Moreover, rough play behavior is not a male trait that depends directly on the presence of a Y-chromosome. Rather, high frequencies of performance of this behavior depend indirectly on the Y-chromosome; i.e., on the secretory products (the androgens) produced by the Y-determined gonad. When genotypic rhesus females are exposed to suitable androgens during the appropriate period of prenatal development, they show rough play postnatally in higher frequencies than normal females (Figure 3). Postnatal treatments of genetic females with potent androgens are ineffective (Joslyn, 1973).

The possibility that the juvenile ovary might actively suppress rough play in normal females has also been studied (Goy, 1970a). It does not, and females ovariectomized on the day of birth show levels of rough play that are not different from those of normal females. Moreover, prenatally androgenized female rhesus monkeys display

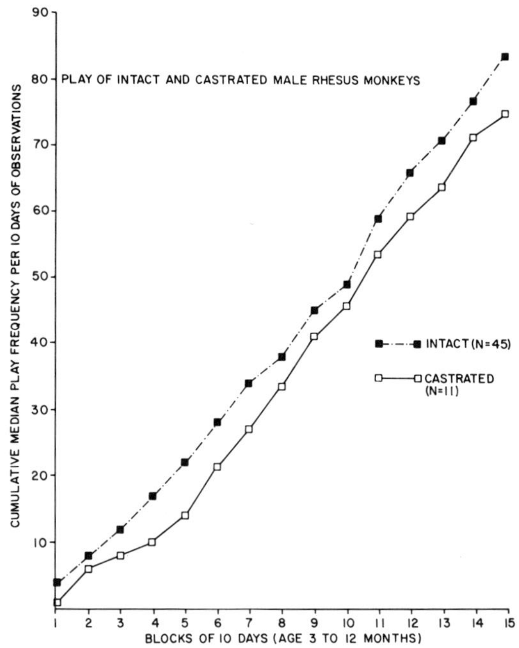

Figure 2. Lack of effect of castration during the first 3 months of postnatal life on the performance of rough play by male rhesus monkeys. [Goy]

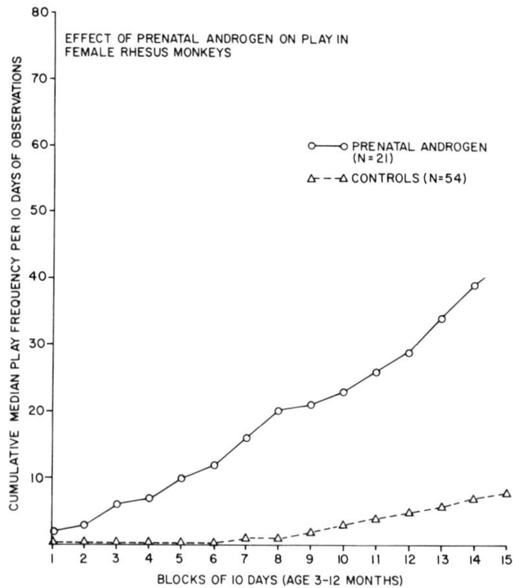

Figure 3. Effect of prenatal androgen on the frequency of performance of rough play by rhesus females during the first year of postnatal life. [Goy]

heightened levels of rough play compared to normal females, although there is nothing discernibly different about their prepubertal ovaries compared with normal females' ovaries.*

Mounting behavior has also been shown to be sexually dimorphic in laboratory studies of juvenile rhesus monkeys (Figure 4). Like rough play, its frequency of performance is unaffected by neonatal castration (Figure 5), and genetic females can be induced to mount significantly more often than controls if they are exposed to androgens prior to birth (Figure 6).

During the juvenile period, mounting behavior is clearly unrelated to reproduction; partners of both sexes are mounted frequently, and the function(s) it might serve is(are) not known. It seems clearly to be a part of the gestural and expressive repertoire, and, as such, some learning of when to mount, whom to mount, and where to mount may

*Unpublished observations from Goy's laboratory.

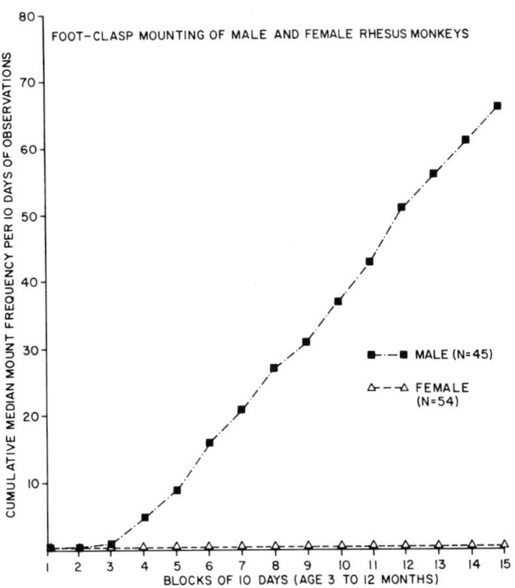

Figure 4. Sex differences in foot-clasp mounting behavior in rhesus monkeys during the first year of life. Note that data are plotted as medians, and the medians for females were never greater than zero despite frequent mounting by a few individual females. [Goy]

be required. The performance of this behavior is very much influenced by social history and testing conditions (Goy and Wallen, 1979). Moreover, the frequency of performance of this behavior can be increased in untreated females by testing them in isosexual (all female) groups (Goldfoot and Wallen, 1978). Isosexually tested females, however, do not become as proficient mounters as control males or prenatally androgenized females.

The reason why females mount only infrequently in heterosexual groups is obscure, but laboratory findings on this point are consistent with those from field studies (Lindburg, 1971). Perhaps the reason is that mounting partly defines the role of more dominant members of the juvenile group. In heterosexual groups of juveniles, the status positions in the upper end of the dominance hierarchy are nearly always filled by male (or androgenized female) members of the group. In isosexual groups, in contrast, only females can be in these higher positions.

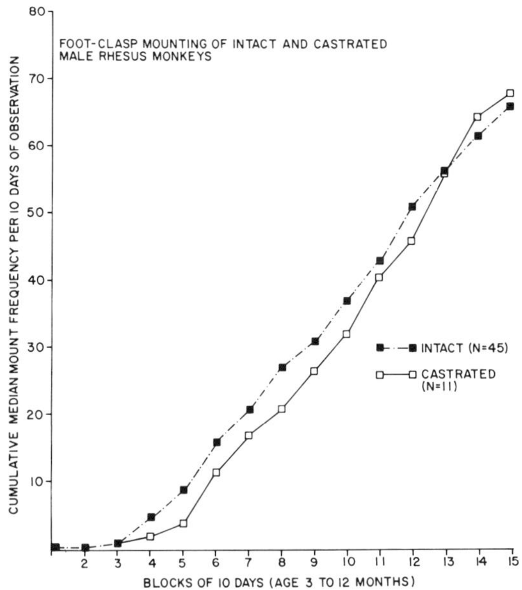

Figure 5. Lack of effect of castration during the first 3 months of postnatal life on the frequency of performance of foot-clasp mounting by male rhesus. [Goy]

Studies of dominance, based on submissive interactions (Goy and Goldfoot, 1974), have been completed recently on six heterosexual groups of rhesus weaned from their mothers at 1 year of age. Five of these groups contained three males and two females and one contained four males and two females. Thus, the groups contained 31 subjects including 19 males and 12 females. Males were ranked alpha in five, and a female was ranked alpha in only one of these six groups. Thus, males achieved alpha more often than chance expectancy (3.67) and females less often than chance expectancy (2.33).

In 18 heterosexual groups of juveniles (studies starting after weaning at 1 year of age) that contained prenatally androgenized females as well as normal subjects, the alpha status was held by males nine times, by prenatally androgenized females six times, and by control females three times. These empirical determinations compare with corresponding chance expectancies of 6.78 alpha positions for males, 4.51 for prenatally androgenized females, and 6.70 for control females.

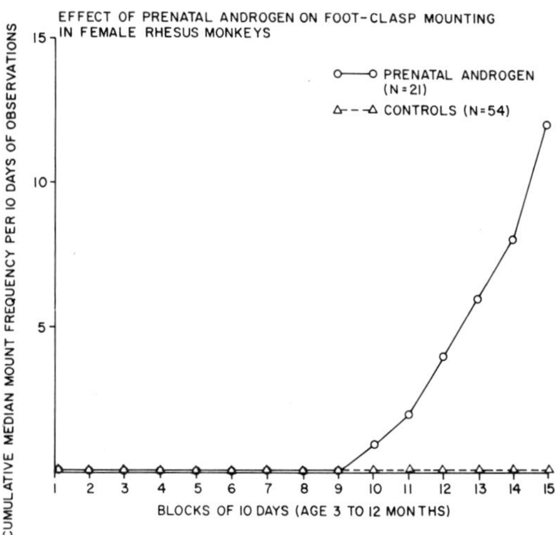

Figure 6. Effect of prenatal androgen on the frequency of performance of foot-clasp mounting by rhesus females during the first year of postnatal life. [Goy]

In summary, in these groups males and prenatally androgenized females held alpha positions more often than expected by chance, and control females held such positions less often. Thus, in laboratory groups that in few respects resemble natural social groups, the tendency of males to hold the higher dominance positions is as characteristic as it is for feral troops. Moreover, prenatal androgenization of the genotypic female produces an individual that is indistinguishable from a normal male in its disposition to high dominance status even when it is studied in a group that contains normal males as peers.

Biological and Environmental Determinants of Sex Differences in Behavior of Humans

Ehrhardt stated at the outset that there are few behaviors in humans that meet the criteria for being called sexually dimorphic, and that among those behaviors where sex differences do exist there is often considerable overlap of the trait distributions for the sexes. Moreover, she stated that the impact of social factors and the environment is presumed to be much greater in humans than even in nonhuman primates. Nevertheless, she believes that it is fallacious to attribute entirely to environmental factors all those sex differences that can be measured.

Ehrhardt lists the following categories of sex differences in human behavior: (1) *sexually dimorphic behaviors* (e.g., maternal behavior) for which one can find somewhat comparable animal models; (2) *cognitive sex differences* (e.g., verbal and spatial abilities) that may have measurable counterparts in lower animals; (3) *gender identity* (i.e., self-identification as male or female, which carries with it the implication of self-awareness) for which there may be no measurable counterpart in other species; (4) *gender role behavior* (e.g., the classification of different games or sports into boys' and girls' activities, or corresponding classifications of adult careers or occupations, e.g., "housewife"); (5) *sexual orientation*, i.e., the choice of a sexual partner (homosexual, bisexual, or heterosexual), for which there is some disagreement among various experts on the existence of animal models.

Whereas it is manifestly impossible, in her opinion, to equate animal behavior with certain human responses (e.g., lordosis in a male rat in response to another male and a man falling in love with another man), it is possible to make some more abstract analogies between behaviors seen in lower animals and in humans and to evaluate effectively biological determinants of some selected human behaviors.

The approach that Ehrhardt, Money, and co-workers have pioneered is based on the measurement of gender identity and a related but independent parameter, gender role behavior, in individuals suffering from congenital or drug-induced abnormalities of body sex differentiation; for example: the androgen-insensitivity syndromes (see Wilson below); *Turner's syndrome* (absence of one sex chromosome and deficiency of gonadal tissue); the *adrenogenital syndrome* (congenital adrenal hyperplasia, *CAH*, or the variety induced by androgenic drugs, such as Provera, given to counteract toxemia in pregnancy) in which there has been some masculinization of reproductive tract, external genitalia, and body type. These conditions are summarized in Table 3, together with the general trend of gender role behavior in such individuals, which is seen to be consonant with endocrine status rather than genetic sex.

Ehrhardt elaborated on this, using as an example the adrenogenital syndrome (CAH). In recent studies, she and Baker (1974) compared CAH females (who were reared as females after surgical correction) with female siblings. These individuals showed higher

TABLE 3

Human Sexual Differentiation [Ehrhardt]

Syndrome	Genotype	Gender Role Behavior	Reference
Turner's syndrome	XO	Feminized	Ehrhardt et al., 1970
Androgen insensitivity	XY	Feminized	Money et al., 1968 Masica et al., 1971
Adrenogenital syndrome	XX	Masculinized	Ehrhardt, 1973, 1977b

activity levels than their siblings, tomboyishness, preference for male friends, and less interest in dolls.

These findings of masculinized gender role behavior in CAH females, in spite of their being reared as females, are particularly striking. Ehrhardt stated that they could find no consistent factors in the mothers' behavior toward affected and nonaffected daughters. Likewise there were no significant birth-order differences between the two groups. Among the CAH females there was a tendency for the most strongly virilized individuals to be the most active and tomboyish. While the exact forms of play that characterize prepubertal male humans and prepubertal male rhesus may not be identical, both of these primates show a clear division of preadolescent activities into gender roles. In both species males show more active and rougher forms of play than females, and the behaviors characteristic of each role may serve comparable functions and may also represent pure homologies. In both species, moreover, females androgenized prenatally assume the male gender role and display its associated behaviors prepubertally. Ehrhardt was then asked whether the higher activity level in CAH females (and also in normal males) might be the primary factor in differences in gender role behavior whereas the other traits, such as preference for male friendships, might be secondary manifestations. She replied that this might be so, but that the fantasies of these children, as manifested in altered patterns of doll playing and rehearsal for marriage and motherhood, could not be accounted for in this manner. Asked about sexual behavior of CAH, she replied that these CAH females were all heterosexual, except for one bisexual individual. A parallel study by Money and Schwartz (1978), with similar observations, led to the conclusion that altered prenatal environment in no way dictates postnatal sexual orientation even though the androgenizing prenatal condition can profoundly alter prepubertal gender role behavior.

An earlier study by Ehrhardt and Money (1967) found that females masculinized in utero by exposure to androgenic progestins showed, as in CAH females, elevated activity levels, preference for male friends, tomboyishness, interest in a career over motherhood, and decreased interest in appearance and doll play.

Besides the effects of adrenal androgens or androgenic progestins in the direction of masculinizing gender role behavior, there are also reports of estrogens and progesterone having the opposite effects, namely, feminization or inhibition of masculinization. Yalom and colleagues (1973) found that males of diabetic mothers exposed to elevated exogenous estrogen prenatally showed lowered aggressiveness and assertiveness and less athletic skill and other kinds of masculine interests, as well as retarded heterosexual development. The finding of estrogenic "feminizing" effects finds some parallels in studies on feminization of male rats by estrogens given shortly after birth (see above) and is not inconsistent with the organizational model described earlier. Estrogens may be acting to inhibit gonadotropin secretion and to interfere with testicular development during differentiation. Results obtained with estrogens are difficult to interpret, however, because these hormones are known to act differently in different species and in some species may have paradoxically masculinizing actions.

In their study of female and male children, aged 16 to 19, of mothers given progesterone (not the androgenic synthetic progestins referred to above) for toxemia in pregnancy, Zussman and colleagues (1975) found lowered physical activity and tomboyishness, and elevated interest in appearance. Ehrhardt and colleagues (1977) studied a comparable situation, girls exposed in utero to medroxy-progesterone acetate vs. matched controls. Though younger (8 to 12 years old) than the children in the Zussman study, these subjects showed a significantly greater preference for feminine clothing styles and a tendency for showing less verbal and indirect aggression, as well as a nonsignificant tendency for lower energy levels, lesser athletic skills, and lesser tomboyishness. It would thus appear that progestins that are not androgenic may counteract androgen effects in utero in females as well as in males. While this is only an hypothesis, there is some support from studies on rhesus monkeys. Resko (1975) found that genetic male and female rhesus fetuses did not differ greatly in terms of the concentrations of circulating estradiol and dihydrotestosterone. Male fetuses, however, had higher concentrations of testosterone in plasma, and females had higher concentrations of progesterone. He argued that the higher concentrations of progesterone "protected" the female fetus from possible masculinizing effects of estradiol and dihydrotestosterone.

In conclusion, Ehrhardt offered three generalizations: First, gender role behaviors, which by definition are different, though overlapping, between males and females, are subject to influences of prenatal hormones and are determined independently of genetic sex, sex of rearing, or of gender identity. Second, gender indentity is always concordant with sex of rearing and is the variable that is most strongly dependent on social environmental factors. Third, the outcome of prenatal virilization or of other disturbances of sexual development is not homosexuality.

Sexual Dimorphism in Human Parenting

Parenting is a behavior that tends to be sexually dimorphic in all mammals owing to the biological factors of pregnancy, birth, and lactation. The study of parenting in humans has been left largely to sociologists and cultural anthropologists who, according to Rossi, have not felt the need to include biological variables to understand and explain this kind of behavior. Rossi is now attempting to inject biological considerations into this kind of research, and, within her specialty of family sociology, discusses sexual coupling, family behavior, pregnancy, mating, and fertility as purely sociocultural phenomena. The strong environmental paradigm is reinforced by the field's sensitivity to feminist issues, oriented toward elimination of sexist assumptions. Yet, we live with the certain knowledge that some sex differences are biological facts; sex equality, in contrast, may be merely a political and social precept. Rossi feels biological scientists are more likely to entertain this possibility than social scientists.

Because of this cultural-deterministic and learning-theory bias in research on human parenting, there have been, thus far, few efforts to confront social science assumptions with the implications of new knowledge in the biological sciences. The belief or assumption by developmental psychologists that gender differences are so structured by social role expectations that real behavioral sex differences can be demonstrated only by the study of neonates disregards the biological data indicating that the hormonal environment for males and females is influenced by maternal hormones postnatally, and different behaviors and bodily functions are only "triggered" at puberty. It also disregards the data relating to dimorphic brain development at critical prenatal periods, which may only result in behavioral differences in early puberty.

Over the past 2 decades the social sciences, in response to the changing sociopolitical climate, have moved away from the study of the parent-child relationship as the core of any family system. Recent research is directed more toward the adult male-female relationship in marriage or sexual partnership. Thus, a special 1972 issue of *The Family Coordinator*, with fifteen articles published on the general theme of "Variant Marriage Styles and Family Forms," actually devotes only 5% of the total 123 full-text pages to any aspect of parenting, child care, or the parent-child relationship (Rossi, 1977a, pp. 13 to 14). Recent research has uncovered and, in turn, been shaped by certain demographic facts of current family life in the United States: (1) families are increasingly small, (2) children are closely spaced, (3) babies are artificially fed, (4) babies are fed and cared for at earlier ages by adults other than the mother as a result of increasing numbers of mothers remaining in or returning to the labor force, (5) single-parent households are rapidly increasing (it is estimated that by 1979 1 in 3 children will be living in homes headed by their mothers), and (6) pressure for child-care facilities is increasing in the United States (but not in Israel, Sweden, and some Eastern European countries, where longer maternal and paternal leave with pay is increasing, or in Czechoslovakia, where there is a trend away from institutional child care for children under 2 years of age). Pressure for child-care facilities is primarily a middle-class and lower-class phenomenon in the United States. Studies of stable working class families show a preference for child care, in the mother's absence, within the family (Woolsey, 1977).

Rossi noted that overall life or marital satisfaction begins to decline with the birth of children, reaches a nadir when children enter adolescence, and improves once the last child leaves home (Rollins and Feldman, 1970; Rollins and Cannon, 1974; Lowenthal et al., 1975; Spanier et al., 1975). The birth of grandchildren, however, is associated with a rise in life satisfaction. An important phenomenon in the U.S. is postpartum depression, which is higher in the U.S. than in any other country. This may be because women are without social support systems (Rossi, 1968; Parlee, 1975); our culture does not allow for the psychological impact of the pregnancy and birth experience, and the medical profession mismanages that experience (Newton, 1963; Arms, 1975; Rossi, 1977a).

Rossi also discussed how the cultural denial of the impact of the birth experience affects sexual dimorphism in parental roles. Such denial, for example, leads to the idea that other care-givers may be readily substituted for the mother. Yet the assumption that fathers can easily function as primary care-givers is not supported by research findings. A study by Fein (1974) of parents who shared natural childbirth training during pregnancy (with fathers present during labor and delivery) indicated that within a few months after birth mothers were more attached to the child than fathers. Studies by Kanter and co-workers (1975) and Berger and co-workers (1972) of communal parenting indicate that, when attempts are made to have multiple care-givers, the children are confused and the mothers show conflict. Generally, within a short period mothers take back many primary care-giving functions. Males tend to be excluded from primary care-giving roles, unless specific sanction is given, until children are about 5 years old. Young children in communes, as in nuclear families, are cared for by mothers and other women; males care for young children only when delegated such duties by the mother.

Female attachment to an infant may be innate, while male attachment may be socially learned. A bioevolutionary perspective argues that the more critical the behavior is to species survival, the more apt behavior is to entail innate, unlearned components. On this basis, one would expect human mother-infant attachment to involve some innate factors, since the female is more directly involved in the reproductive process than the male, and there is greater need for close bonding of the human infant than for other members of the species (Blurton-Jones, 1972; Hamburg, 1974). Human mothers tend to cradle their infants in their left arm, regardless of their particular handedness, where the children can be soothed by the maternal heartbeat familiar from uterine life; close-up films of women after childbirth indicate strong attempts on their parts to establish face-eye contact with their infants. Infant crying stimulates oxytocin secretion in the mother that triggers uterine contractions and nipple erection preparatory to nursing. Females show pupil dilation when shown pictures of a baby while males do not. These and other research findings are consistent with the theory that there are two innate orientations to the female—one involving sexual attraction to men and the other a care-giving attachment to the child—while the male has only the innate sexual attraction to the female and learns most parenting behavior from females (Washburn and Dolhinow, 1972; Count, 1973).

Elevated hormonal levels during pregnancy and birth may be implicated in mother-infant attachment, according to Rossi, and the attachment process is both dyadic and two-directional. From their research, Stern (1974), Klaus and co-workers (1970, 1972), and Leifer (1970) all suggest that early physical contact immediately after birth has long-lasting impact on the quality of maternal investment in the infant. Recent evidence also suggests that constitutional characteristics of the child affect this process (Lewis and Rosenblum, 1974). A good example is seen in child-abuse research. Where it was long thought to be exclusively parental pathology that accounted for abuse of children, recent evidence suggests that excessive fussing, strange and irritating crying, and other exasperating behaviors on the part of the child can trigger abusive reactions not only from parents, but from foster parents and even researchers (Gil, 1970). Robson and Moss (1970) have reported that the attachment of mothers to their babies weakened by the end of the third month if the baby's crying and fussing did not decrease according to the pattern of most infants by that age. Thus, there is a growing suggestion in this literature that neurological or hormonal factors in the infant may contribute to the attachment process with the maternal care-givers.

No known society replaces the mother as the primary care-giver. For example, Whiting (1963; Whiting and Whiting, 1974), in a study of child rearing in six cultures, found that it is confined to adult women or pubescent girls; this is similar to most nonhuman primates. Males, on the other hand, tend to become interested in the young only as they mature.

Life-span research in sociology has yielded a profile of sexually dimorphic behavior throughout life that reveals relatively few strong sex differences in prepubescence. However, sex differences increase rapidly during adolescence and early adulthood and wane in late-middle and old age. According to Lowenthal (1975), older women become more assertive and confident while older men display softened, more nurtural qualities. The consequence of these age-related changes is a lessening of sex differences, and this fact raises questions regarding the explanation that sex differences are exclusively based on social training and sex role expectations. Long decades of reinforcement and training have preceded the blurring of gender differences in old age. The increased hormonal differentiation of the sexes beginning in puberty and its lessening in the postmenopausal and postclimacteric years are a more "efficient" explanation than the socialization theory commonly offered by social scientists. Reinforcement and learning theories are not powerful explanatory concepts for the menopausal gender reversals in behavior and personality.

The "naturalistic" observation of parenting in humans, if it is to be reflective of a social structure for which humans were designed over the course of 99% of our history, has to be carried out in hunter-gatherer societies. Dramatic changes in the political and cultural systems of modern society, compared to most of our history as humans, blur and distort the expression of innate sexually dimorphic behaviors, including parenting. Lee (1965; Lee and DeVore, 1968, 1976) studied the !kung bushmen and found their parenting dramatically different from parenting in modern societies. Mothers have a high level of physical contact with infants: 70% of the day compared to 25% in modern families, falling to 30% by about age 2½ for the !kung child, compared to 5% in our culture. There is virtually continuous rather than periodic nursing, and lactation is continuous until the child is 4 to 5 years of age. There is a close, indulgent emotional relationship between mother and infant with wide birth spacing of almost 4 years. By age 2 to 3 the child gradually shifts his center of activity to a multiage heterosexual play group. This pattern seems typical of most primate species living in groups of over 25 individuals. The most important implication of this pattern is that Westernized human beings not living in a technological world are still genetically equipped only with an ancient mammalian primate heritage that evolved largely through adaptations appropriate to the hunter-gatherer type societies that characterized 99% of human history.

The development of a settled agricultural society, only about 12,000 years old, created dramatic changes in child rearing. For example, birth rates increased and average birth spacing decreased. This resulted in a less close mother-infant relationship, with maternal aides and shorter lactation periods. Moreover, peer groups were segregated by sex and later by age.

There are also changes resulting from 20th-century technological advances: (1) modern obstetrics replaced natural childbirth in a family setting (for research on effects see Klaus and co-workers (1970, 1972)); (2) short-term bottle feeding replaced long-term lactation; (3) the mother-infant pair is socially isolated most of the time. Problems in the "socialization" of children and in mothering may, in fact, be signals of stress resulting from environmental demands alien to our biological needs. Such stresses include separation of mother and infant in the hours immediately following birth when hormonal levels are still high. This period may contribute uniquely to the attachment of the mother and infant. Coupled with the much lower amount of bodily contact and tactile stimulation during infancy, this could engender a disruptive discontinuity with the behavioral biology of the human species. In stepping outside the known range of reaction of the human species, we may expect stress signals as inevitable consequences. Thus, the drastically lowered rate of body contact during infancy due to the use of cribs, strollers, clothing, and bottle feeding may have important effects on the developing infant and the affectional and attentional investment of parents in the child. We know that low levels of stimulation can affect the development of close emotional relationships on which early learning is dependent. So, too, the change in human sleeping patterns due to changes in family structure and household design may be implicated in such problems as difficulties in going to bed, crib death, children's nightmares, and the 2-year old's fear of strangers. Similarly, narrowing of the age spacing between children may disturb and reduce the degree of parental investment in the individual child. Obviously, cause and effect between the changes occurring in human life-style and the problems of children have not been proven by these observations. Nevertheless, sociologists ought not to regard their association as mere coincidence on the one hand, or as totally unrelated to the biological consequences of altered social patterns on the other hand.

The issues above affect precisely the major three areas accepted as differentiating the sexes: lactation, pregnancy, and childbirth. Modern social and technical interventions, by departing radically from a pattern held for most of human history, have tended to minimize sexual dimorphism in precisely these fundamental aspects of human life, thereby potentially interfering most profoundly in the process of mother-infant attachment. There are few research themes more in need of collaborative work by both biological and social scientists than these areas critical to human welfare. In Freud's day, the key concepts were those such as cathexes, repression, and sublimation. In the heyday of behavioral psychology, it was stimulus-response connections. In the future, we may learn that beneath the behavioral manifestations of mother-infant attachment, neurochemical processes and neuroactive molecules provide a substratum that facilitates that attachment, but only if social and technological inventions do not distort their proper functioning.

Is There an Endocrine Basis for Homosexuality Among Human Males?

Theories of the origins of homosexuality, and of sexual orientation more generally, either focus on the role of prenatal (or perinatal) influences of sex hormones on the brain (Dörner, 1977) or of postnatal learning, i.e., of psychosocial influences on behavioral development (Ehrhardt, 1977b). These two variables need not be conceptualized as mutually exclusive, however, and the possibility that they accomplish their effects best by working in concert is definite.

Dörner bases his work upon a vast literature, to which his laboratory has contributed significantly (Dörner, 1972, 1976, 1977). Male rats castrated on the first day of life showed predominantly heterotypical behavior following androgen substitution in adults. In other words, genetic males exposed to a temporary androgen deficiency during sexual differentiation and maturation of the brain, but normal or approximately normal androgen levels in adulthood, were sexually excited preferentially by partners of the same sex. The higher the androgen level during a critical differentiation phase, the stronger was the male and the weaker the female sexual behavior during the post-puberal functional phase, irrespective of the genetic sex. Even a complete inversion of sexual behavior was observed in male and female rats following androgen deficiency in males and androgen excess in females during sexual differentiation of the brain.

According to these findings, a neuroendocrine predisposition to primary hypo-, bi-, and homo-sexuality may be based on different degrees of androgen deficiency in males and androgen excess in females during sex-specific brain differentiation. Furthermore, in adult male rats castrated on the first day of life, a strong positive estrogen feedback effect could be induced in a similar way as in normal females, but could not be induced in males castrated on the fourteenth day of life or in neonatally androgenized females. In view of these findings, a positive estrogen feedback effect appeared to be evocable only if a low androgen level existed during brain differentiation.

In addition, the following correlations between sex hormone levels during the period of differentiation and the evocability of a positive estrogen feedback effect on LH secretion were observed in rats (Figure 7): Following a single estrogen injection in postpuberally ovariectomized and estrogen-primed females, a distinct surge of luteinizing hormone (LH) secretion was evoked, while ovariectomized

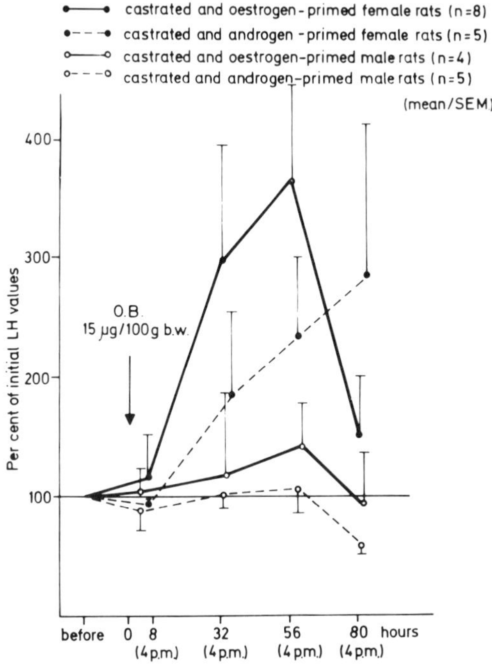

Figure 7. Serum LH response to a subcutaneous injection of estradiol benzoate (OB) (15 μg/100 g body weight (b.w.)) expressed as percent of the mean initial LH values in postpuberally castrated and estrogen- or androgen-primed female and male rats. [Dörner]

and androgen-primed females displayed a diminished and delayed increase of LH secretion. On the other hand, postpuberally castrated and estrogen-primed males exhibited only a slight but significant increase of LH secretion, whereas castrated and androgen-primed males did not display any increase of LH secretion following estrogen injection. In view of these findings the evocability of a positive estrogen feedback action on LH secretion appears to be dependent on the sex hormone level during both a critical differentiation phase that occurs neonatally in rats as well as during the postpuberal period.

Investigations carried out on humans revealed the following data (Dörner et al., 1975b; Dörner, 1976, 1977): a positive estrogen feedback effect could be elicited in homosexual men in contrast to heterosexual and bisexual men (Figure 8). Thus, in homosexual men, an intravenous injection of estrogen (20 mg of Presomen, which is comparable to Premarin) produced, primarily, a decrease of the LH serum level followed, secondarily, by a significant increase above the initial LH serum level. On the other hand, in heterosexual and in

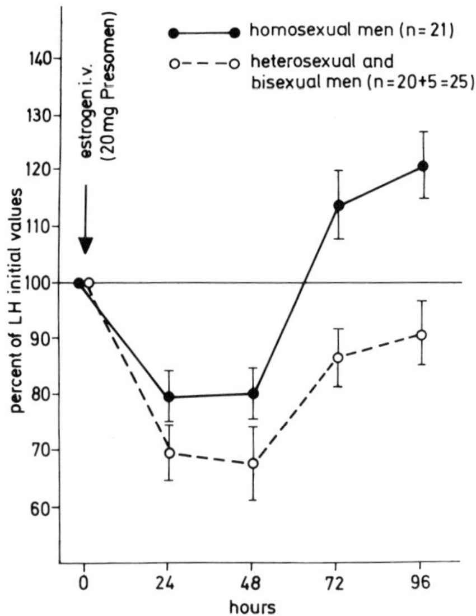

Figure 8. Serum LH response to an intravenous estrogen injection expressed as percent of the mean initial LH values in homosexual and heterosexual or bisexual men (mean ± S.E.M.). [Dörner]

bisexual men, the estrogen administration also produced a decrease of the LH serum level that was not followed, however, by an increase above the initial LH values. These findings suggest that homosexual men may possess, at least in part, a predominantly female-differentiated brain, possibly based on androgen deficiency during brain differentiation.

More recently, the plasma basal levels of free and total testosterone as well as of FSH and LH were determined in homosexual and heterosexual males (Stahl et al., 1976; Dörner , 1977; Rohde et al., 1977). As shown in Figure 9, significantly lower free plasma testosterone levels were found in effeminate homosexual males than in heterosexual males. In contrast to free testosterone levels, no significant difference of total plasma testosterone levels was observed between homosexual and heterosexual males.

As Figure 10 shows, significantly higher plasma FSH concentrations were found in effeminate homosexual males and transsexual males

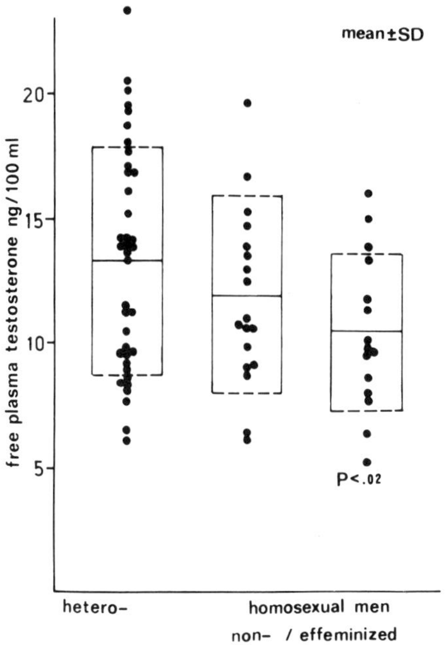

Figure 9. Free plasma testosterone levels in heterosexual and noneffeminized or effeminized homosexual men. [Dörner]

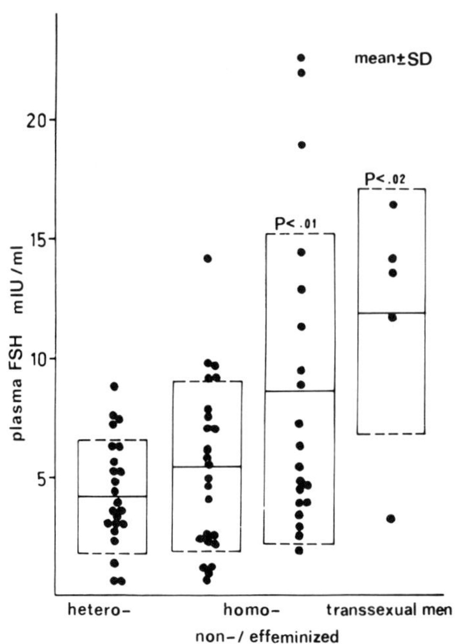

Figure 10. Plasma FSH levels in heterosexual, noneffeminized or effeminized homosexual, and transsexual men. [Dörner]

as compared to heterosexual males. Significantly higher plasma LH concentrations were also observed in homosexual males, particularly in effeminate homosexuals, and in transsexual males as compared to heterosexual males (Figure 11).

In view of these experimental and clinical data, the following working hypothesis was deduced: an androgen deficiency occurring in genetic males during prenatal life might give rise to predominantly female differentiation of the brain. This prenatal androgen deficiency can be largely compensated by increased hypophyseal gonadotropin secretion in postpuberal life. However, an approximately normal androgen secretion by means of increased gonadotropin secretion may be achieved only by a simultaneous slight increase of estrogens. Increased plasma estrogen levels were found, indeed, in homosexual males (Doerr et al., 1976). An increased estrogen level, in turn, leads to increased binding capacity of the sex hormone globulin, resulting in a

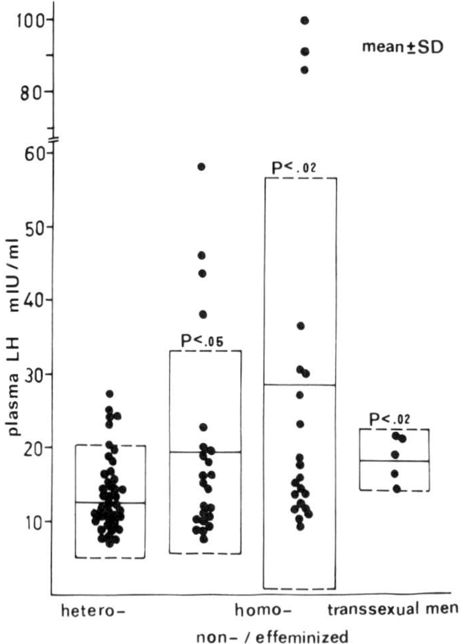

Figure 11. Plasma LH levels in heterosexual, noneffeminized or effeminized homosexual, and transsexual men. [Dörner]

decreased percentage of plasma-free testosterone (Rohde et al., 1977). Thus, the predominantly female-differentiated brain is exposed postpuberally to a slightly decreased (but normal ranged) free androgen level and a slightly increased estrogen level. This endocrine profile is associated with homosexual behavior. Note that identical postpuberal endocrine conditions could be experimentally induced in heterosexual males without leading to homosexual behavior because of presumed differences in brain differentiation.

Hence, according to Dörner, psychosexual orientation in humans may be based, at least in part, on discrepancies between the genetic sex and the sex-specific sex hormone level during brain development in prenatal life. Therefore, methods were developed for the determination of genetic sex and sex-specific sex hormone levels in amniotic fluids in order to detect and possibly to correct such discrepancies in prenatal life.

The cell nuclei in amniotic fluid cells of genetic male fetuses show a brightly fluorescing Y chromosome after staining with quinacrine—a phenomenon successfully used for the determination of genetic sex (Dörner, 1972, 1976). As shown in Figure 12, testosterone glucuronide (TG) as well as unconjugated testosterone (T) levels were found to be significantly increased and FSH levels significantly decreased in amniotic fluids of male fetuses as compared to those of female fetuses between the sixteenth and twenty-sixth week of pregnancy (Clements et al., 1976; Dörner, 1972, 1976; Dörner et al., 1977b). Therefore, according to Dörner, the examination of amniotic fluids for genetic defects could be supplemented in the future by the determination of hormone levels in order to find abnormalities that might lead to altered processes of differentiation, especially of the brain. First of all, however, male fetuses with lower than normal testosterone levels as well as female fetuses with higher than normal testosterone levels in amniotic fluids should be followed up with respect to their sexual development in postnatal life.

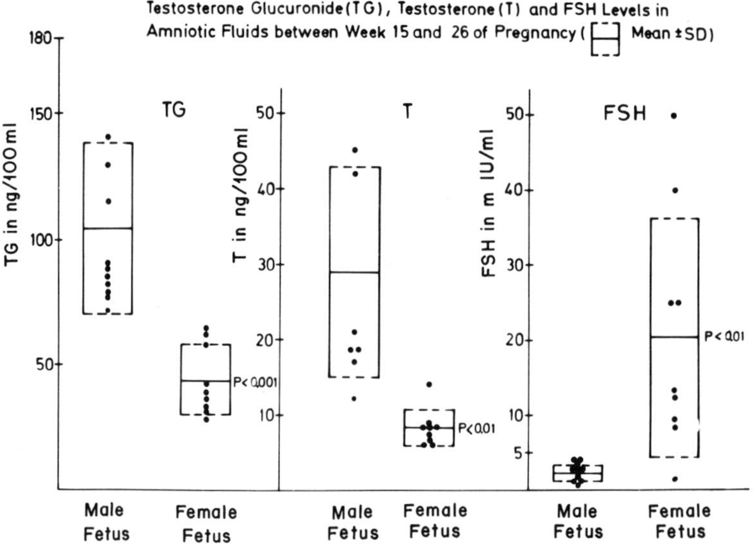

Figure 12. Testosterone glucuronide (TG), unconjugated testosterone (T), and FSH levels in amniotic fluids between weeks 15 and 26 of pregnancy. [Dörner]

Dörner believes the evidence is strong enough that, to prevent development of sexual disturbances, androgens are completely contraindicated in pregnant women carrying female fetuses, while antiandrogenic substances are contraindicated in pregnant women carrying male fetuses. Unphysiologically high estrogen doses should also be avoided during pregnancy. In cases of adrenogenital syndrome, especially in female fetuses, glucocorticoid treatment should be started prenatally in order to inhibit adrenal overproduction of androgens. Moreover, adrenal or ovarian tumors producing sex hormones should be removed in early pregnancy. Furthermore, preventive therapy of sexual differentiation disturbances, if desirable at all, might also become possible in the future by administration of androgen in genetic male fetuses with clear-cut evidence of androgen deficiency during critical differentiation periods.

Dörner's findings evoked considerable discussion, centering around the probable cause of the rise in LH after estrogen. A LH rise has also been observed after estrogen treatment in castrated male rhesus monkeys (Karsch et al., 1973) and in castrated human males (Dörner et al., 1975a; Kulin and Reiter, 1976). Such a positive estrogen feedback effect, however, was found only in estrogen-primed male primates, as it was also observed in estrogen-primed but not in androgen-primed male rats (Figure 7). Furthermore, prenatally androgenized female rhesus monkeys showed ovulatory cycles in later life, unlike perinatally highly androgenized female rodents. However, systematic studies in monkeys with planned variations in dosage and duration of prenatal androgen treatment are in progress (Goy et al., 1977). Even female rats androgenized as late as the tenth day of life—unlike those androgenized on the third day of life—show ovulatory cycles in later life associated with strong heterotypical behavior (Dörner and Fatschel, 1970). This finding suggests a time-dependent partial dissociation between the differentiation periods of central nervous "sex centers" regulating gonadotropin secretion and "mating centers" responsible for sexual behavior (Dörner, 1976).

Ovulatory cycles can also be induced by glucocorticoid treatment in prenatally androgenized women with congenital adrenal hyperplasia. Such cycles, however, can disappear again in spite of continued treatment (Trampuž, 1968).

Returning to the alternative hypothesis, namely, that homosexuality is a learned condition, it was pointed out again—referring to

Meyer-Bahlburg (1977)–that partially successful behavior therapy approaches to changing sexual orientation would make the learning hypothesis particularly attractive. In this context, however, Marmor and Green (1977) have stated: "The majority of adults neither seek nor desire therapy, and the majority of those who do seek therapy continue to remain homosexually oriented. In general, those homosexuals who are younger, below 35 years of age, who are less feminine, have had their first overt homosexual experience after the age of sixteen, and who give a history of some potential for heterosexual arousal, have a better prospect for achieving some sexual reorientation so as to include some degree of heterosexuality. The same type of change may occur developmentally, without treatment."

In view of recent findings of Dörner's group (1976, 1977), neurotransmitters appear to represent, as local hormones of the brain, common mediators of systemic hormones (e.g., sex hormones) and of psychosocial influences as well. Thus, both abnormal levels of sex hormones and abnormal psychosocial influences–if occurring during critical periods of brain development–might lead to permanent alterations of sexual behavior and orientation. Therefore, theories of hormonal and psychosocial influences on sex-specific brain development and sexual orientation might be no longer mutually exclusive alternatives but, rather, complementary.

Clearly, immense philosophical differences exist among workers regarding the validity, usefulness, and desirability of the hypothesis that is being examined in this section. The notion that the selection, choice, or differential erotic responses to partners on the basis of their sex could be established independently of experience is difficult for many to conceive. At the same time, there is a great willingness on the part of these same critics to acknowledge that some biological factor independent of, or in addition to, experience probably contributes to selection of sexual role and sexual partner.

There are, however, major empirical obstacles to be overcome before this hypothesis of an endocrine determination of homosexuality can gain wider acceptance. Not the least of these is that an accounting of the disorder by use of the concept of a critical period cannot be accomplished without an empirical demonstration of such a period. Such a period would have to begin after genital differentiation had already occurred; otherwise, genital defects would accompany the psychosexual variation. Moreover, endocrinopathies that result in male genital abnormalities would also be associated with homosexuality if their critical periods coincided. Another empirical obstacle is the lack of any convincing spontaneous or experimental animal model for homosexuality. We are not surprised at unique human characteristics that are based on culture or experience, but there is an expectation (justified or not) that biological phenomena can be duplicated in some other species. Still other deficiencies in the amount and kind of empirical evidence needed for acceptance of the hypothesis were voiced by other participants at the Work Session. Their repetition here serves no particular purpose beyond emphasizing the consensus that much more evidence is needed. Let us all recognize the fact, however, that the hypothesis is here and cannot be dismissed.

III. GENETIC ASPECTS OF SEX DIFFERENCES IN BEHAVIOR AND SEXUAL DIFFERENTIATION

General Considerations

According to Manning, progress in behavioral genetics has been restricted by the intractable nature of much behavior for genetic analysis. We know a good deal about the microevolution of behavior and can understand how small quantitative behavioral changes result from mutation and recombination. We know little of how the potential to perform the basic repertoire of sexual behavior patterns is encoded in genetic terms (see Manning, 1975, 1976).

The pathway through which genes control sexual differentiation is: chromosomes→gonads→hormones→brain, and these steps will be elaborated in detail in a later section. Because of the large number and dispersed nature of the genes affecting sexual behavior, both male and female must inherit bisexual potential. The problem for natural selection has thus been how to make the sexes different; hence, the operation of hormonal switches has become widespread. It must be recognized that as we concentrate on mammals we are seeing only one type of sexual development amongst many. There are many and diverse patterns of sexual differentiation and development through the vertebrates. Some fish, for example, can change their sex and gender role according to the requirements of their social and physical environment (see "Introduction" above). Many invertebrates are hermaphroditic or parthenogenetic.

The main steroid hormones must be phylogenetically very ancient—as old as the vertebrates—and evolution has involved their target organs more than the hormones themselves. There is, as the earlier sections of this volume have documented, a great variety of nonsexual behaviors that differ between the sexes, e.g.: maternal behavior, rough-and-tumble play, aggression, and locomotor activity. Many of these can be shifted in the male direction in mammals by pre- or post-natal androgenization.

Although evidence is not yet fully adequate, Manning considers the Adkins (1975, 1977) hypothesis on the comparative sexual differentation of the vertebrates to be promising. The sexual pattern of the homogametic sex (female in mammals, male in birds) will differentiate unless the heterogametic patterns are "switched in," as it were, by the action of gonadal steroids from the heterogametic gonads. Even then, the homogametic sex retains a greater degree of bisexuality: it is generally easier to elicit masculine responses from the female mammals and the converse in birds. There are exceptions, such as the bisexuality of the male hamster, which can display good lordosis behavior as well as homotypical mounting and copulation. As with any biological hypothesis that attempts a broad generalization, exceptions must be expected. Natural selection will achieve adaptation in diverse ways according to circumstances; or, as Charles Phoenix would say: "It's the exception that proves there is no rule."

Many fixed-action patterns are involved in sexual behavior, and these appear to be governed by many genes that are dispersed through the genome. The contribution of the Y chromosome is apparently small because relatively few effects have been linked to it. Certainly the most obvious and important is the determination of the sex of the gonad (Mittwoch, 1970). Another indication of Y-chromosome involvement in one type of sexually dimorphic behavior derives from the work of Ginsburg's group (Selmanoff et al., 1975). They have shown by reciprocal crosses between inbred mouse strains that the Y chromosome has an important effect on the level of aggression shown by males. This result has recently been confirmed by Stewart and co-workers (1979) using the C57BL/b and CBA strains.

In human males, there is a distinct increased risk of antisocial behavior (possibly aggressive behavior) among individuals carrying the XYY chromosomal complement (Meyer-Bahlburg, 1974). Thus, aggression does seem to be associated with the Y chromosome in some mammals, with the likelihood that other chromosomes are involved as well. We do not know the mechanism of this involvement—whether it is an influence on hormone secretion, on brain structure and function, or on something entirely different.

Manning described a number of techniques that are useful for the genetic analysis of behavioral traits associated with hormones and with sexual differentiation. One of these is the analysis of genetic mosaics, which is possible in mice, using the X-linked *Tfm* gene, which causes androgen insensitivity. Ohno and co-workers (1974) have constructed mosaic mice, originally female, which are heterozygous both for the sex-reversing X chromosome gene *Sxr* and for *Tfm*. Since one of the X chromosomes in every cell will be inactive, the brains of these animals will consist of a mosaic of neurons carrying *Tfm* (and therefore insensitive to androgen) and normal neurons. Different individuals of such phenotypic males exhibit a wide variety of sexual behavior, but it is quite clear that a mouse does not need anything like 100% fully functioning androgen-sensitive neurons to display adequate male behavior. There is obviously a good deal of redundancy at the neuronal level, which is familiar enough with vertebrates. Ohno and co-workers could also demonstrate that the neurons responsible for sexual behavior are distinct from those controlling aggression.

Another approach to the genetics of sexual behavior involves the use of recombinant inbred lines (Bailey, 1971). Here an F_2 population derived from crossing two inbred lines, contrasted in sexually dimorphic behavior, is subjected to brother-sister mating. If a reasonable number of such lines can be established, different loci affecting the behavior become fixed in some of them. With enough lines one may hope to be able to identify some of the more obvious genes affecting behavior. Eleftheriou and co-workers (1974) have used this method and have located two loci with major effects on male aggression. The method has its uses but requires the facilities of a Jackson Laboratory if more than a tiny and random sample of loci involved are to be isolated.

Although there are some exceptions, and always bearing in mind the possibility that hormones and experience may be interchangeable in the activation of sexual behavior, it is, nevertheless, a useful generalization that, as an evolutionary trend, the higher on the phylogenetic scale, the less rigid is the dependence of sexual behavior upon hormones. As McGill and Tucker (1964) first pointed out, it is not sufficient to judge the hormone dependence of rodents from the behavior of inbred lines (see also McGill, 1970). Among inbred strains of mice, where dependence of sexual behavior on hormones is usually strong, there is at least one example of a genetically based independence from them. The sexual behavior of male F_1 hybrids between two inbred lines C57BL/6 and DBA/2 (the B6D2F_1) shows a remarkable resistance to castration and adrenalectomy (McGill and Manning, 1976; Manning and Thompson, 1976; Thompson et al., 1976). Other F_1 hybrids do not show the same resistance, and their sexual responsiveness may be just as much affected by the withdrawal of testosterone as that of their parental inbred lines (McGill and Manning, 1976). It is unlikely that neonatal castration will completely abolish the sexual responsiveness of B6D2F_1 males, as even normal hybrid females display mounting and intromission-like responses (Manning and McGill, 1974). In short, there is a particular genetic combination in $B6D2F_1$ mice that renders activation by gonadal steroids less necessary. The instatement of this program is presumably facilitated by perinatal androgen secretion, but not entirely dependent upon the androgens secreted during the brief postnatal period only. Prenatal androgens, for both the female and the male, probably play some role. Moreover, since $B6D2F_1$ males show more independence from activational androgens than $D2B6F_1$ males (the reciprocal cross), some contribution from the maternal (C57BL/6) environment, or the maternal X chromosome, or both is suggested (McGill and Manning, 1976).

There is another example of a genetically controlled behavioral difference, the manifestation of which is under control of neonatal androgens. Male mice of Balb/c strain are more aggressive than males of the A or C57BL/6 strains; females are not aggressive, but Balb/c females given 1 mg of testosterone propionate on day 3 of life are moderately aggressive and much more aggressive than androgenized females of the other two strains (Vale et al., 1972). In other words, inherited strain differences in aggression that are latent in the genetic female are developed and revealed when the brain undergoes sexual differentiation according to the male pattern. Similarly, strain differences in mounting behavior by females show heritability. $C57BL/6F_1$ females mount frequently when injected with TP in adulthood whereas DBA/2 females do not. Hybrids ($D2B6F_1$) show intermediate frequencies (Holman, 1976).

Androgen-Insensitivity Syndrome: Behavioral Aspects

One of the most successfully studied disorders involving genetic control of hormonal sensitivity is the androgen-insensitivity (AI) syndrome. In the complete androgen-insensitivity syndrome in humans and in a comparable syndrome in rats and mice, the primary defect is the virtual absence of androgen receptors (discussed below by Wilson); this results in feminine body traits. Both developmental and activational effects of androgens are severely deficient in AI individuals; i.e., there can be a complete failure of masculine development of the Wolffian duct, urogenital sinus, and external genitalia and a severe deficiency of sensitivity to activational effects of androgen in the kidney, salivary glands, and brain.

With respect to the brain and neuroendocrine and behavioral effects of androgens, there are a number of studies on the AI rat (Naess et al., 1976; Beach and Buehler, 1977). In spite of normal or above-normal androgen levels in blood, AI rats have high blood levels of LH and FSH that increase only slightly or not at all after castration, compared to normal controls in which intact blood levels are low and the postcastration increase is marked. This indicates a deficiency of negative feedback mechanisms in the AI rat. Administration of low doses of dihydrotestosterone propionate (DHTP) (50 μg) failed to suppress LH and FSH in AI rats but did so in normal castrates, whereas high doses of DHTP and TP (2 mg) did exert some suppressive effects on LH and FSH in the AI rat. The authors explain this latter observation by noting the existence of a small number of androgen receptors in target hypothalamic tissues of the AI rats (Naess et al., 1976).

AI male rats show a general deficiency in all components of male sexual behavior, although they are clearly able to display such behavior (Beach and Buehler, 1977). This and the fact that lordosis behavior in the AI rat is as poor as it is in wild-type males have been interpreted as follows: ". . . in AI males . . . central neural mechanisms involved in mediation of male behavior are normally organized but markedly insensitive to testosterone; and . . . mechanisms responsible for manifestations of feminine behavior are like those of the normal male in their relative lack of responsiveness to estrogen and progesterone" (Beach and Buehler, 1977). Data supporting these observations and obtained from AI mice have been reported by Shapiro and co-workers (1976) and by Ohno and colleagues (1974). In these experiments, displays of both male and female behavior by AI mice were very poor. Further support for the masculine tendency of the brain of AI rodents is provided by experiments in which ovarian grafts in castrated AI rats failed to show indications of ovulatory cycles, thus resembling the status of grafts in castrated wild-type males (Shapiro et al., 1975). Yet AI rats also show feminine-type saccharin preference, and so the masculinization is not complete (Shapiro and Goldman, 1973).

The predominantly masculine state of the AI rodent brain may be due to two factors: Either the small number of androgen receptors in the AI brain is sufficient to permit sexual differentiation to occur or the pathway of sexual differentiation involves a mechanism independent of androgen receptors. Because of the evidence cited below for the role of the aromatization of testosterone, McEwen tends to favor the second possibility. In this connection it has been demonstrated that androgen receptor levels in the AI mouse brain are, at most, 10% of normal, but brain estrogen receptors are undiminished (Attardi et al., 1976). On the other hand, the role of androgen receptors in brain sexual differentiation cannot be totally discounted. There are the reported antagonistic effects of an antiandrogen, cyproterone acetate, on brain sexual differentiation (Neumann and Steinbeck, 1974). Cyproterone acetate does prevent androgen interaction with cerebral androgen receptors (Lieberburg et al., 1977) but may have other effects, including inhibition of aromatization (Schwarzel et al., 1973).

Whatever the mechanism whereby the AI rodent brain acquires masculine character, this occurrence appears to be different from the human complete AI syndrome, in which there is no evidence whatsoever for masculine tendencies in gender role behavior. This suggests a primary role for androgen receptors in human brain sexual differentiation and is supported in another primate species by the finding that both T and 5α-dihydrotestosterone (DHT, a nonaromatizable androgen) cause masculine sexual differentiation when given prenatally to female rhesus monkeys (Goy, 1978).

Ehrhardt elaborated on human androgen insensitivity in relation to two other genetically based disorders of hormone production and/or sensitivity: Turner's syndrome and the adrenogenital syndrome (CAH), which was discussed earlier. In the complete form of AI, there is a feminine appearance, strongly feminine attitudes toward marriage and maternalism, and satisfaction with gender of rearing, which in every case was female (Money et al., 1968; Masica et al., 1971). The AI individuals showed predominantly normal female sexual orientation and reported, for the most part, having experienced orgasm. In contrast, CAH girls and women show masculinized attitudes toward marriage and maternalism, and other features of gender role behavior are also in the masculine direction (see earlier comments of Ehrhardt). Turner's syndrome, which involves the absence of one sex chromosome and streak ovaries with little or no active ovarian tissue, results in feminine gender role behavior and a sexual orientation concordant with the sex of rearing (which, incidentally, is never male).

There is one indication that AI individuals may not have entirely escaped from the influences of testicular secretions on development. Using an estrogen treatment regimen able to induce a normal LH surge in normal women, Aono and co-workers (1978) were unable to demonstrate a similar LH rise in normal males and in AI males. The reasons for these results in genetic males remain in the realm of controversy, for the reader will recall that in the discussion of homosexuality (see above) it was noted that castrated human males and nonhuman primate males can show an LH surge in response to estrogen treatment. Given the apparent lack of androgen sensitivity in human AI subjects, the only route for circulating androgens to exert effects antagonistic to LH discharge would be through the pathway involving conversion to estrogens.

There is an unusual form of incomplete androgen insensitivity reported several years ago by Imperato-McGinley and colleagues (1974) in which there was delayed development of the phallus (so-called "penis at twelve" syndrome). These individuals appear to lack the enzyme 5α-reductase rather than the androgen receptors. There is considerable disagreement over the gender identity of these individuals. The authors claim that these children shifted from a female sex of early rearing to a male sex role at adolescence. However, Ehrdhardt argues that this may not have been the case at all, and that such individuals appear now to be raised as males from birth onwards. Furthermore, the fact that these cases were well known in their small village in the Dominican Republic and that they lived in different cultural circumstances makes evaluation very difficult. Ehrhardt cited two cases of incomplete androgen insensitivity in which sex of rearing was female. Even though virilization of the phallus occurred at puberty, there was no reversal of the gender identity (Imperato-McGinley and Peterson, 1976). However, the cases cited by Ehrhardt clearly have a more profound insensitivity to androgen, as evidenced by extensive perineal-scrotal hypospadias, than the cases in the Dominican Republic.

IV. CELLULAR AND MOLECULAR ASPECTS OF SEXUAL DIFFERENTIATION

Introduction

It will be recalled that many aspects of sexual differentiation of birds and mammals differ with respect to the pattern, male or female, that predominates when gonadal secretion is absent during the critical period. Yet many aspects of the sexual differentiation process in birds and mammals are so similar that they deserve to be treated together. The following discussion treats birds and then mammals with respect to sexual differentiation of the gonads and reproductive tract and then deals with morphological sex differences in mammalian and avian brain and their possible cellular origins.

In the context of sexual differentiation, the critical period is defined as the time during which a tissue is most sensitive to the developmental (also called organizational) effects of hormones. A number of interrelated factors must be considered: (1) the period when gonadal secretion normally occurs in the genetic female bird or genetic male mammal and (2) the maximum period of susceptibility of the tissue (e.g., reproductive tract, brain) to the action of the hormone. Experimentally, this is determined by removing gonads at various ages and by hormonal treatment.

Sexual Differentiation of Gonads and Reproductive Tract of Birds in Relation to Genetic Sex

The genetic constitution of male birds in regard to sex chromosomes is ZZ and that of females is ZO. The assumption that Z in the female has no small partner was confirmed by the study of meiotic divisions in the spermatocytes of a sex-reversed hen (Miller, 1938). A single Z moves ahead of other elements to one pole of the first meiotic spindle; it has no partner going to the opposite side. According to Nottebohm, a very useful review of the genetics, anatomy, and physiology of sexual differentiation in birds is found in Witschi's article (1961). Witschi suggests that: "Genetic interpretation leads to the assumption that each Z chromosome carries a male-determining gene or gene complex (M) which is quantitatively balanced against female-determining genes (FF) in another chromosome pair in such a way that ZZ (2 M) assures male differentiation, ZO (1 M) female differentiation."

The embryonic avian gonads are composed of three kinds of elements: *medulla* (of mesonephric origin); *cortex* (modified peritoneal wall); and *germ cells* (of endodermic origin). Testicular differentiation results from a prevalence of medullary development and the reduction and eventual disappearance of the cortex. In ovarian differentiation, the cortex is the leading element. A parsimonious interpretation of sexual development is that ZZ inhibits cortical development, leading to the formation of a testis. ZO fails to suppress cortical development, and cortical development, in turn, suppresses medullary (testicular) development.

Sexual differentiation in avian embryos occurs toward the end of the first half of the incubation period. The gonads of male embryos may temporarily exhibit an ambisexual character, being covered by more or less extensive cortical crusts. These remnants usually disappear before hatching. During ovarian development medullary remnants may persist in various structural forms (Witschi, 1935). Under certain circumstances these remnants may later enlarge and become the source of hermaphrodite development and sex reversal. So, for example, genetic females may suffer sex reversal after pathologic regression of the ovarian cortex, as reported in domestic fowl. In two instances hens that had been laying eggs changed into cocks, each one fathering two offspring before their death (Crew, 1923; Arnsdorf, 1947).

Normally, female birds develop only one ovary, the left one, a mere gonadal rudiment persisting on the right side. Benoit (1923) was the first to report that removal of the left ovary in hens leads to anatomical and behavioral masculinization. Removal of the left ovary is followed by a compensatory hypertrophy of the right rudiment, which in most cases assumes a testicular function (Domm, 1939). Similar observations have been reported for ducks (Cavazza, 1938), though not for passerines. Witschi (1961) interprets these observations as revealing "a persistent antagonism between (gonadal) cortex and medulla."

Steroid hormones are known to influence sexual development in female birds. Following a first announcement by Kozelka and Gallagher (1934), it became widely established that all estrogens produce a temporary feminization of gonad differentiation in genetically male embryos (Dantchakoff, 1941; Willier, 1942; Et. Wolff, 1950). Intriguingly, though, these early experiments also report a gradual reversion to the male sex within the first year after hatching (see also Boss and Witschi, 1947). The classical work of Em. Wolff (1950) and Wolff and Wolff (1949) on the development of the phallic tubercle and the syrinx in ducks suggested almost 3 decades ago that at least some aspects of avian male conformation represent "neutral" type, i.e., the type that will develop in the absence of gonadal influences. Their basic observation was that the tubercle and syrinx acquire a typical male conformation in early castrates of either sex. Even rudiments grown in vitro, removed from gonadal influences before the ninth day of incubation, assume the male-type characteristics. Addition of estrogens to the culture media results in the development of female-type characteristics (Wolff, 1952). At puberty the phallic organ of male ducklings becomes a large penis under the influence of testicular hormones, and this mature male condition does not regress after castration but retains a nearly constant adult size (Benoit, 1936). Thus, a male trait can become manifest in the absence of gonadal hormones, then further develop under the influence of androgens, and retain this final condition despite subsequent castration.

Sexual Differentiation of Gonads and Reproductive Tract in Mammals

There are a number of generalizations that can be made regarding sexual differentiation in mammals: (1) The timing of the critical period is unrelated to the time of birth and may occur prenatally in some species, postnatally in others. In two species, rat and guinea pig, the critical period occurs at similar chronological ages from conception, even though birth occurs before the critical period in the rat and after it in the guinea pig. (This point is discussed earlier by Goy.) (2) The reproductive tract undergoes its critical period somewhat before the brain, although there is temporal overlap. Various aspects of brain sexual differentiation (e.g., male, female sexual behavior, aggressive behavior) must be regarded as separable events–temporally, as well as in terms of the kinds of hormones that influence them, and the degree to which they may be influenced at all in a given species (this point is discussed above and below).

According to Weisz, definition of the exact time and duration of the period critical for the sexual differentiation of the developing brain in different species has been limited by the fact that, unlike the situation in the anlage of the secondary sex structures, no obvious, easily identifiable, immediate structural and functional changes have been recognized to mark the differentiating action of androgens on the CNS. Rather, investigators had to depend on observation of the long-term, remote functional and structural consequences of manipulations of the hormonal environment during fetal or neonatal life. Thus, information on the *total duration of the critical period* during which the CNS is maximally responsive to the differentiating effects of testicular hormones has been deduced from observing, generally after puberty, changes in ovulatory function and/or behavior resulting from exposure of the female to androgens during early development. The duration of the critical period has, in fact, been delineated by this approach in only very few mammalian species. In their early pioneering studies, Phoenix and co-workers (1959; Goy et al., 1964) showed that behavioral masculinization occurred in female offspring only in mothers treated with testosterone during the fifth week of pregnancy. Brown-Grant and Sherwood (1971) confirmed these findings in other strains of guinea pigs. These investigators also observed the effects of the androgen treatment on cyclic ovarian function, the end point generally used to identify the differentiating action of hormones on gonadotropin regulation. They found days 33 to 37 postconception to span the critical period for masculinization of gonadotropin release, indicating a substantial overlap with the critical period for masculinization of mating behavior.

There are important ongoing studies of the phenomenon of sexual differentiation in the nonhuman primate, in particular the rhesus (Goy, 1970; Resko, 1974). In this species, the critical period appears to span a relatively long time at least from days 40 to 60 of pregnancy.

The sheep is the third mammalian species in which systematic studies have been carried out to delineate the duration of the period of vulnerability of the fetal CNS to androgens (Clarke et al., 1976a,b, 1977). The pregnant ewes were implanted with testosterone for various periods of time. Ovulation, estrous behavior, and urination pattern were then examined in the female offspring as adults. As this study demonstrates, it is easier to reach a conclusion about when the critical period ends than when it begins. Estrous behavior could be modified till about 70 to 80 days of gestation and the urination pattern until 80 to 90 days. According to the author, "the results are complicated to interpret because androgen appears to act on the fetal brain over an extended period of time rather than at one critical instant." The expectation that the task would prove easier may have been due to the fact that many of our concepts on the sexual differentiation of the CNS have been derived from observations on the rat. In this species, major modifications of CNS structure and function can unquestionably result from hormonal manipulations restricted to a brief postnatal period (Harris, 1964). However, as discussed below, even in the rat the critical period spans a considerably longer period of time than such observations would lead one to suppose, and androgen acts on the developing brain of the male over an extended period of time.

Our knowledge of when, within the overall critical period, masculinization takes place in normal males of different species is even more limited. For information on this point we have had to depend, to date, primarily on experiments involving surgical or chemical castration of the male. The paucity of data on this point is not surprising. In most mammalian species, masculinization of the CNS is completed prenatally. Surgical manipulations on fetuses in utero are not easy to carry out, and truly satisfactory chemical agents for surgical castration have not been available. In those species in which the young are born at a relatively immature stage in their development, such as the rat, mouse, and ferret, the process of normal CNS masculinization extends into the postnatal period. For reasons of convenience, therefore, many investigators have focused their attention on the postnatal phase of sexual differentiation in such species, in particular the rat.

In the rat, the species most frequently used in studies of the sexual differentiation of the mammalian CNS, the critical period clearly extends into the postnatal period, as does the period during which normal males undergo androgen-dependent changes in CNS differentiation (Harris, 1964). Males castrated on the day of birth exhibit substantial deficits in male sexual behavior as adults and can respond like females in the mating situation if pretreated with the appropriate hormones. They can as adults also maintain cyclic ovarian function with ovarian implants and presumably can release LH in response to estradiol (Harris, 1964; Neill, 1972; Brown-Grant, 1973). Masculinization and defeminization of sexual behavior and of gonadotropin regulation do not appear to be completed for several days after birth. An increased potential for female sexual behavior and a decrease in male behavior are exhibited even in rats that have been castrated as late as day 5 postnatally (Grady et al., 1965; Gerall et al., 1967), and ovarian cyclicity can be maintained in ovaries transplanted into adult male rats of some strains castrated as late as day 8 postpartum (Marić et al., 1974). However, there is a great deal of evidence that the critical period during which the CNS of the female rat is vulnerable to the differentiating action of androgens begins in utero, as does the normal process of masculinization in the male. This fact, though often ignored, becomes evident when reproductive behavior is examined in greater detail. Although neonatally castrated male rats can exhibit female mating behavior when treated with the appropriate hormones, this behavior is qualitatively and quantitatively inferior to that of the normal female (Gerall et al., 1967). Thus, androgen in utero appears to have already blocked some of the potential for female sexual responses. This conclusion is confirmed by the observation that prenatal androgen inhibits the sexual receptivity of female offspring (Gerall and Ward, 1966; Nadler, 1969; Ward and Renz, 1972), and by the finding that males exposed to the antiandrogen, cyproterone acetate, are already prenatally more completely feminized than those treated only postnatally (Ward, 1972). Conversely, females given androgen only postnatally show deficits in male copulatory behavior, the full development of which requires the action of androgen in utero (Nadler, 1969; Ward, 1969, 1972; Ward and Renz, 1972; Sachs et al., 1973). Completion of the organization of the neural substrate required for the ejaculatory response occurs under the influence of testosterone postnatally (Nadler, 1969; Sachs et al., 1973).

The question of whether there are components of the gonadotropin regulatory mechanism in rats vulnerable to masculinization before birth has been examined less closely. The development of anovulatory sterility apparently cannot be achieved easily by exposing females to testosterone prenatally. At best, a delayed anovulatory syndrome could be achieved in a few of the female offspring that had been exposed prenatally, via maternal injection of testosterone, to sufficient androgen to masculinize the external genitalia (Swanson and van der Werff ten Bosch, 1965; Adams-Smith, 1970). More substantial disruption of female gonadotropin regulation might be achieved if the steroid is introduced into the amniotic fluid (Fels and Bosch, 1971).

In agreement with the concept of the prenatal onset of the normal process of sexual differentiation in rats is the observation that there are sex differences in the volume of cell nuclei in the medial preoptic area and the ventromedial nucleus that become statistically highly significant between day 20 of gestation and the day of birth (Dörner and Staudt, 1969a,b). It is reasonable to assume that the action of testosterone must have preceded this event by some period of time. The importance of testicular androgens before day 20 for the normal process of CNS masculinization is suggested also by the finding that the most consistent and greatest sex differences in plasma testosterone concentrations in rats occur on days 18 and 19 of pregnancy. Furthermore, it is only on days 18 and 19 that plasma testosterone levels are significantly lower in male rat fetuses of mothers who have been exposed to a regimen of stress that results in failure of behavior masculinization in their male offspring (Ward and Weisz, 1977).

There are several conclusions that may be drawn from the studies cited above, besides the most obvious one, that even in the rat, there is an important prenatal component to the normal process of male sexual differentiation of the CNS. These are as follows:

1. *Within what may be termed the overall critical period there appear to be periods of special sensitivity, i.e., distinct critical periods for different components that make up the total, normal pattern of response.* These have been defined to some extent in the rat with respect to behavior. A comparable critical examination of gonadotropin regulation may well reveal a similar phenomenon in relation to this function as well. The "end points" used as markers of CNS function need to be examined in detail when trying to evaluate the consequences of early hormonal manipulations and delineating "critical periods."

2. *Potentially important differences in neuronal organization may underlie superficially similar functional states.* This principle is illustrated by a few studies and applies to the control of gonadotropin release as well as of behavior (Taleisnik et al., 1969; Södersten, 1976). For example, Taleisnik and co-workers (1969) have demonstrated that progesterone can facilitate LH release in long-term castrated female rats following priming with either estradiol or testosterone, but will do so in long-term castrated males only after testosterone priming. The neonatally androgenized female differs from both of the above. Gonadotropin release in such females is facilitated by progesterone only after estradiol pretreatment. The neonatally castrated male, on the other hand, though feminized in some respects, responds in this test situation as does the normal male. This is one of the very few studies in which the gonadotropin-releasing mechanism was investigated in such detail.

In most other studies, the abolition of cyclic ovarian function was equated with masculinization. Only in a few was even the integrity of the estrogen positive feedback mechanism also tested.

3. An additional important point, illustrated by the studies of Taleisnik and co-workers (1969), is *the potentially disruptive effect of excess androgen in the male during critical developmental stages.* Exogenous testosterone given to male rats during the neonatal period abolished their ability as adults to respond with acute gonadotropin release to progesterone after testosterone priming. In several behavioral studies, it was also noted that excess testosterone during early development diminished rather than augmented normal masculine sexual behavior (Sachs et al., 1973; Baum and Schretlen, 1975).

Thus normal masculine differentiation would appear to require not only that the appropriate steroids be present but also that they be in the circulation for the requisite period of time and in the correct amounts. Within this context, it is of interest to note that much of the differentiation of the CNS appears to occur, at least in rats, during the period when circulating testosterone levels in the males are actually declining (Weisz and Ward, 1979). A more complete understanding of how the fetal testes control normal masculine differentiation of the CNS would require additional knowledge of how the circulating levels of hormones in fetuses vary during the whole of the duration of the critical developmental period in different species.

Since our information on the exact timing of the critical period for CNS differentiation is limited to a few species and even in these it is incomplete, it is probably premature to try to make any generalizations at this time such as, for example, the stage of general development when it is likely to occur. However, from observations made on the four species in which the critical period for CNS differentiation has been studied, it would seem that it occurs after the initiation of sexual differentiation of the urogenital ridge and accessory organs of reproduction, although the two processes may overlap to a considerable degree as, for example, in the guinea pig. Clearly, a much more precise definition of the exact timing of the critical periods for the differentiation of the various sexually dimorphic, CNS-mediated functions is needed before it is possible to evaluate the hormonal milieu optimal for normal sexual differentiation. This information is also required for basic studies of the process of androgen-dependent CNS differentiation.

Testicular Development and Circulating Testosterone Levels in Relation to the Critical Period of Sexual Differentiation of the Mammalian CNS

Although testosterone is considered to be the major hormonal determinant of sex differences in CNS-mediated functions established in mammals during the fetal and/or perinatal period, we have little information on the levels of this crucial androgen in the circulation during the stage in development that is presumably critical for sexual differentiation of the brain. A key problem, discussed earlier, is our imprecise knowledge of the period of time during which the developing brain of different mammalian species is vulnerable to the differentiating action of testosterone or when, during this time, masculine differentiation normally takes place in the genetic male.

In every mammalian species examined so far, it has been possible to show unequivocally that the fetal testis can synthesize and secrete testosterone early in its development. It has also been shown in a few species that the mean levels of testosterone in the circulation of males are higher than those of females, at least during a certain period in fetal development. However, this information on circulating androgen levels cannot be related to the process of masculine differentiation of the CNS until we know when this is actually taking place. This question is crucial when trying to identify the etiology of disturbances in normal sexual differentiation of the CNS and certainly before it is possible to contemplate any therapeutic intervention. As discussed elsewhere, normal masculine differentiation may not depend simply on the presence or absence of testosterone during a particular period of time but probably also on the brain's being exposed to amounts of androgen appropriate for each particular stage in its development. There is evidence that too much testosterone at the inappropriate time may be disruptive not only to normal sexual differentiation of the female but also to that of the male (Sachs et al., 1973; Baum and Schretlen, 1975).

Steroidogenesis by the fetal testes and, more specifically, their capacity to synthesize and secrete testosterone have been studied in a number of mammalian species. However, investigators were generally interested in the role of the developing testes in masculine differentiation of the urogenital ridge and in establishing correlations between these two functions. Certain features that may have greater relevance to the sexual differentiation of the CNS than to that of the accessory organs of reproduction, such as development of the testicular vasculature, have received scant attention. Clearly, to act on the brain, the androgens produced by the fetal testes must reach the systemic circulation in adequate concentrations, while they may reach the urogenital ridge by local diffusion (Jost, 1965). In the adult testes the interstitial cells are characteristically clustered around capillaries. This is not seen in the early stages of testicular development in the rat (Roosen-Runge and Anderson, 1959).

Testosterone and Rat and Guinea Pig

The rat and the guinea pig are the two species for which we have the most detailed information both on the timing of the critical period of CNS masculinization and evidence on the development of the androgen-producing potential of the testes. Numerous aspects of the steroidogenic function of the rat fetal testes have been examined by a variety of approaches. Exact correlations between the different studies are at times impossible, since different strains were used and because in some cases the method of dating the pregnancy was not specified. In the rat the testes can synthesize and secrete testosterone in vitro as early as day 14½ postconception (pc) (Price and Pannabecker, 1956; Noumura et al., 1966; Warren et al., 1975; Picon, 1976; Feldman and Bloch, 1977; Sanyal and Villee, 1977). The onset of testicular testosterone production coincides with the appearance of Δ^5-3β-ol-steroid dehydrogenase in presumptive Leydig cells in the interstices between the seminiferous tubules (Niemi and Ikonen, 1961; Schlegel et al., 1967; Lording and De Kretser, 1972). The potential of the testes in vitro to produce testosterone, whether from endogenous precursor or from those supplied in the incubation medium, increases sharply after 14½ and plateaus around 18 to 21 days pc (Noumura et al., 1966; Warren et al., 1975; Picon, 1976; Sanyal and Villee, 1977). This correlates well with data on plasma testosterone levels, which are highest in male rat fetuses on days 18 to 19 pc and decline thereafter (Weisz and Ward, 1979). Testosterone synthesis and secretion by the testes appear to occur even before it is possible to identify cells in the interstitium with the structural features that are considered, in the adult, to be characteristic of the steroid-producing cells (Narbaitz and Adler, 1967;

Lording and De Kretser, 1972; Merchant-Larios, 1976). Typical Leydig cells with well-developed, smooth endoplasmic reticulum appear after day 17 pc and become abundant by day 18 (Merchant-Larios, 1976). We thus have to assume that before day 17 testosterone is produced by precursors of these typical Leydig cells—cells with a rich ribosomal population more typical for embryonic and undifferentiated cells than for steroidogenic ones (Palade, 1955; Grasso et al., 1962; Duck-Chong et al., 1964). The appearance of typical Leydig cells after day 17 also appears to coincide with increased vascularization of the testes (Merchant-Larios, 1976). Around the same time there may also occur some changes in the utilization of precursors by the Δ^5-3β-ol-steroid dehydrogenase enzyme system reflected by a greater ability to utilize pregnenolone in addition to dehydroepiandrosterone (Lording and De Kretser, 1972). Between days 14½ and 21 pc, there is also a progressive increase in the ability of the fetal testes to respond to LH with an increase in testosterone secretion in vitro (Picon, 1976; Feldman and Bloch, 1977; Sanyal and Villee, 1977).

Masculine differentiation of the urogenital system in the rat appears to correlate with the first phase of rising testosterone-producing potential of the fetal testes between days 14½ and 17½ pc. Stabilization of the Wolffian duct system is considered to be completed around day 17 pc; i.e., at the time when regression of this duct system is completed in the female (Stinnakre, 1975) and when the concentration of testosterone in the urogenital ridge of the male is maximal (Bloch et al., 1975).

There has been only one report to date on the levels of LH in the circulation in rat fetuses. According to Choudhury and Steinberger (1976), plasma LH and FSH concentrations are high on day 16 pc in male rat fetuses but undetectable in female littermates. These observations correlate well with sex differences in pituitary morphology that have been identified in rat fetuses. According to Yoshimura and coworkers (1970), the cellular differentiation of what they consider to be precursors of the cells that secrete gonadotropins is more advanced in males than females from day 16 pc. The basis for these sex differences in gonadotropic function at this early stage in fetal development is not clear. According to current understanding, it should be hormonal. However, in the two sets of pooled plasma samples from 16-day-old fetuses (representing up to 5 litters each) no sex differences were found in plasma testosterone levels (Weisz and Ward, 1979).

After day 16, plasma gonadotropin concentrations decreased sharply in males, reaching the same low levels in both sexes postpartum (Choudhury and Steinberger, 1976). During the late fetal stage a reciprocal feedback relationship appears to exist between the testes and the anterior pituitary. Decapitation of the fetus or compression of the brain with paraffin reduces Leydig cell volume, while intrauterine castration is cited as causing an increase in the percent of pituitary basophils (Eguchi et al., 1975).

The concentration of luteinizing hormone-releasing hormone (LHRH) in the hypothalamus of rat fetuses was measured by two groups of investigators (Eskay et al., 1974; Araki et al., 1975). In the first of these studies some LHRH was detectable by day 18 pc, in the second only by day 1 postpartum. Unfortunately, LHRH in male and female hypothalami was not separately measured.

The guinea pig is the second species in which there are adequate data on both the timing of the critical period of CNS differentiation and on the development of the testes. The studies were carried out on different strains and therefore the timing of developmental events might not be fully comparable. The female fetus has been found to be most responsive to the masculinizing effect of testosterone on gonadotropin regulation between days 33 to 37 pc (Brown-Grant and Sherwood, 1971) and on behavior between days 30 to 37 (Goy et al., 1964). Morphological differentiation of the urogenital duct is considered to begin around day 29 and to be completed by day 38 (Price et al., 1967). On day 29 pc, Δ^5-3β-ol-steroid dehydrogenase first becomes detectable in the testes (Ortiz et al., 1966). Testosterone secretion can be detected, however, by explants of testes from fetuses as young as 25 day pc (Brinkman, 1977). The amount of testosterone secreted during the first 24 hours in tissue culture increases progressively with testes obtained from older guinea pigs, reaching a maximum around days 29 and 30 pc. There are morphologically readily identifiable interstitial cells in fetal guinea pig testes by days 27 to 30 (Black and Christensen, 1969). These cells contain smooth endoplasmic reticulum but are described as also bearing scattered clusters of ribosomes, suggesting an intermediate stage in differentiation.

Androgens in Mammalian Fetal Circulation

Although the data in the preceding section on the development of the testes and of their steroid secretory potential in different species are of obvious interest, to understand the implications of these findings for androgen-dependent differentiation we need to know the levels of the relevant androgens, testosterone in particular, reaching the brain. Testosterone has been measured in the fetal blood in a number of species and at different stages in pregnancy. In addition, amniotic fluid has been assayed for its testosterone concentration. Hormone concentration in the amniotic fluid may be considered to reflect the amount of androgen excreted by the fetus and, therefore, indirectly, its circulation levels (Resko, 1970, 1975; Kim et al., 1972; Abramovich and Rowe, 1973; Resko et al., 1973; Challis et al., 1974; Giles et al., 1974; Meusy-Dessolle, 1974; Reyes et al., 1974; Mongkonpunya et al., 1975; Payne and Jaffe, 1975; Pomerantz and Nalbandov, 1975; Veyssi et al., 1975; Judd et al., 1976; Belisle et al., 1977; Dawood and Saxena, 1977; Dörner et al., 1977b; Kunzig et al., 1977; Pirani et al., 1977; Robinson et al., 1977; Warne et al., 1977; Zondek et al., 1977).

The general picture that emerges is that in all species there is, at some early stage of development, a period during which circulating testosterone levels are, in general, higher in males than in females. This, however, is not sustained. How the peak levels of testosterone relate to sexual differentiation of the CNS cannot be evaluated, since we have little or no information on the timing of the events in the CNS for most of the species for which we have sequential data on plasma testosterone levels. As indicated previously, this has been established with some degree of accuracy only for the guinea pig, rat, rhesus monkey, and sheep. Therefore, at this stage, only data on circulating testosterone levels in fetuses from these four species can serve to further our understanding of the relevance of the changes in the level of this key hormone to the process of CNS masculinization.

Surprisingly, there are no data on androgen levels in fetal guinea pigs. Yet, this is one species in which both the beginning and the end of the critical period have been defined with some degree of precision (Phoenix et al., 1959; Goy et al., 1964; Brown-Grant and Sherwood, 1971) and in which the fetuses are large enough to provide sufficient blood for hormone measurements without having to pool too many individual samples. Published data on testosterone levels in fetal rhesus monkeys are only from the period after the presumed critical period, although measurements are now being made on blood obtained from earlier stages, i.e., before day 50 (Resko, 1974).

A systematic study of plasma testosterone levels in rats encompassing the period critical for the sexual differentiation of the CNS, from day 17 through the first postnatal day, has been completed in a collaborative study between Weisz and Ward (1979). A puzzling aspect of their findings is the substantial overlap in plasma testosterone values of male and female fetuses and neonates. Also surprising is the number of instances in which testosterone levels in plasma pools obtained from males and females from the same litter(s) were comparable or in which the values of the females actually exceeded those of the males. This was seen on each day of pregnancy with the notable exception of day 18 pc. Testosterone levels in the males appeared to peak on days 18 and 19 pc, with mean values reaching over 2000 pcg/ml. They fell thereafter to around 1450 pcg/ml by day 21 pc. Plasma testerone levels in females throughout this whole period were surprisingly high, with means ranging from about 1000 to 1400 pcg/ml, and similar to those reported by Turkelson and co-workers (1977) for 21-day-old female rat fetuses. Thus, absolute differences between plasma testosterone levels after day 19 were relatively small. The sex differences in plasma testosterone concentrations were highly significant on day 18 pc ($P = <0.005$) and were maintained, in spite of the overlap in individual values, through day 21 ($P = <0.05$ to 0.025). The finding of these surprisingly high testosterone levels in the circulation of the female rat fetus and the substantial overlap in values between the sexes necessitate a careful check on the specificity of the radioimmunoassay used. When using an antiserum to measure hormones, specificity of the antibody cannot be guaranteed. It is only possible to test the specificity of the antibody against known hormones. Similarly, it is only possible to devise separation techniques for hormones that have been already identified. It is a reasonable assumption that there are still a goodly number of unidentified steroids in the circulation, some of which may cross-react with the antibody and which may not be separated by the standard chromatographic systems. In the study by Weisz and Ward (1979), these pitfalls were guarded against by using a number of different antibodies, six in all, developed against testosterone conjugated at different points on the steroid molecule and using different chromatographic systems. Similar values were obtained with all the antibodies and with different chromatographic techniques. Therefore, at this time we have little reason to suspect that a steroid other than testosterone was being measured.

The fall in circulating plasma testosterone values after day 19 pc correlates with the decrease in relative amounts of Leydig cells in the developing testes during the last days of fetal life described by Roosen-

Runge and Anderson (1959) and by Lording and De Kretser (1972). Progesterone concentrations or testosterone to progesterone ratios in plasma of female fetuses did not differ significantly from those of males in the study by Weisz and Ward (1979). This is in contrast to the findings in the rhesus monkey in which progesterone has been proposed as an agent protecting the female from androgenization (Resko et al., 1973).

The lack of a consistent or large sex difference in testosterone levels in rat fetuses from the same litters during much of the period when sexual differentiation of the CNS may be assumed to be taking place challenges some of our basic assumptions. One possible explanation that deserves consideration is that the elevated levels of testosterone in males on day 18 and possibly day 19 pc prime the system so that masculinization in the males can thereafter proceed with testosterone levels not very much higher than those of females. This priming event could involve induction of nuclear estrogen receptors or, perhaps, the aromatizing enzyme system in discrete areas of the CNS.

The hypothesis that adequate concentrations of testosterone need to reach the brain of male rate fetuses around days 18 and 19 for CNS mechanisms regulating mating behavior to develop along normal masculine lines is supported by the findings of circulating testosterone levels in fetuses whose mothers have been exposed to a regimen of stress that results in failure of behavioral masculinization in male offsprings. Plasma testosterone concentrations were significantly reduced in male fetuses of these mothers only on day 18 pc.*

For comparison and for evaluating the significance of these findings in the rat for other species, the only available data are those on sheep. At least the end of the critical period has been defined for sheep, and there is also some information on testosterone levels, although data on the important period, before day 80, have been obtained on fetuses from the slaughterhouse. Therefore, the dating of fetal age was based only on crown-rump length and is consequently only approximate.

Comparison of these data from different publications on the sheep suggests that sex differences in plasma testosterone concentrations in this species may be greater than in the rat at some phase of the critical period; but, as in the rat, testosterone levels are decreasing rapidly during the final stages of the critical period (Pomerantz and

* I.L. Ward and J. Weisz, unpublished observations.

Nalbandov, 1975; Clarke et al., 1977). However, no definitive comparisons are possible until testosterone levels are measured in sheep fetuses from dated pregnancies and of the same strain as the ones used in studies of the period of vulnerability of the female to the effects of exogenous testosterone.

The most important determinant of sexual differentiation of the brain, according to our current understanding, is testosterone, the major androgen secreted by the testes and the agent primarily responsible for carrying the message of the genetic sex to the CNS. Progesterone is of importance by virtue of the fact that it can act as an antiandrogen (Kincl and Maqueo, 1965; Diamond, 1966). To this list of hormones important for CNS differentiation, we must add the estrogens, since the evidence for their role in masculinization of brain, at least in rats, is now rather convincing (see below). Furthermore, if estrogen is the ultimate androgen in this situation, then agents that can protect the brain from circulating estrogens, i.e., plasma steroid-binding proteins (Raynaud et al., 1971), or agents that can modulate the conversion of testosterone to estradiol in brain, e.g., progesterone (Naftolin et al., 1975b), need to be considered as important variables. Then, the placenta, the primary source of progesterone, and the liver, the source of circulating binding proteins, need to be considered, in addition to the testes, as organs that play a direct role in influencing sexual differentiation of the CNS.

Reproductive Tract Differentiation in Mammals

In the rat the temporal aspect of androgen secretion as discussed by Weisz can be described in relation to reproductive tract differentiation as described by Wilson. According to Wilson, the process of masculine differentiation of body sex is imposed by testicular secretions on developing tissues that would otherwise acquire the feminine phenotype (see Figure 13). This process consists of two components: regression of the Müllerian ducts and masculinization of the Wolffian ducts, the urogenital sinus, and the urogenital tubercle and swelling. All of this occurs in the rat from approximately the 16th postconception day until the first or second day after birth. Müllerian duct regression is regulated by an unidentified testicular hormone, possibly a peptide

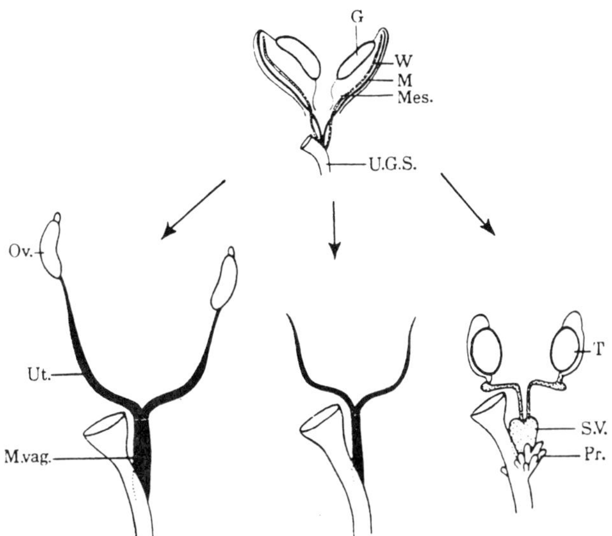

Figure 13. Schematic presentation of sexual differentiation of the sex ducts in the rabbit fetus. From the undifferentiated condition (*top*) may arise either the female structure (*lower left*), the male structure (*lower right*), or the feminine gonadless structure in castrated fetuses of either sex (*lower middle*). G = gonad; M = Müllerian duct; Mes = mesenephoros; Mvag = Müllerian vagina; Ov = ovary; Pr = prostate; SV = seminal vesicle; T = testis; UGS = urogenital sinus; Ut = uterine horn; W = Wolffian duct (stippled). [Jost, 1961]

(Josso et al., 1975). The transformation of the Wolffian duct into epididymis, vas deferens, and seminal vesicles, the induction of prostate development from the urogenital sinus, and the differentiation of the urogenital tubercle and swelling into the male genitalia are all caused by testicular androgens. In the rat, as in most mammals, it appears to be testosterone that stimulates Wolffian duct development and a testosterone metabolite, 5α-dihydrotestosterone, that stimulates development of the urogenital sinus and external genitalia (Schultz and Wilson, 1974; Goldstein and Wilson, 1975). Evidence for this generalization is that DHT formation precedes virilization in the urogenital sinus and external genitalia and follows virilization in the Wolffian ducts. It should be noted, however, that the receptor system mediating virilization of the Wolffian ducts does respond to high doses of DHT in the rat (Schultz and Wilson, 1974).

Reproductive Tract Development in the Human: Genetically Based Defects and Aspects of Mechanism

The differential role of T and DHT leads to an important difference between two forms of androgen insensitivity in humans (Goldstein and Wilson, 1975). Wilson's laboratory has extensively studied reproductive tract development in humans using a variety of hereditary defects of androgen action, including incomplete and complete pseudohermaphroditism. These mutations occur in XY individuals, all of whom develop normal testes with normal androgen secretion rates; but, for a variety of reasons, these individuals are resistant to their own testicular secretions and their phenotypic differentiation is incomplete. These four disorders, summarized in Table 4, are endocrinologically, phenotypically and genotypically distinct.

As noted above, there are, in the development of the normal male reproductive tract, at least three hormonal principles that are responsible for the translation of genetic sex into phenotypic sex: (1) the Müllerian regression factor; (2) testicular testosterone, which is required by the Wolffian duct for its development prior to its ability to convert T to dihydrotestosterone; and (3) DHT, formed locally from T, which is required for the virilization of the urogenital sinus and the urogenital tubercle to form the prostate and external genitalia, respectively.

Proof of this scheme comes not only from timed sequence studies in embryos but also from studies of pseudovaginal perineoscrotal hypospadias in the human (Type 2 in Table 4). To understand this, we have to turn to the model of testosterone's intracellular action shown in Figure 14 (Wilson, 1976a). In this scheme, T enters the cell probably by diffusion, then is converted to DHT. DHT binds to a protein receptor molecule, and this steroid-receptor complex becomes "activated." The activated complex then enters the cell nucleus and interacts with specific acceptor sites on the chromatin, resulting in transcription of dormant genes ultimately affecting the phenotypic expression of that cell. In Type 2 there is normal Müllerian duct degeneration and normal Wolffian duct stimulation, including the presence of a normal epididymis, as well as the presence of other Wolffian duct structures – vas deferens, ampulla of vas deferens, and ejaculatory duct. These individuals also have normal testes and yet have female external genitalia. In examining tissues from these individuals, there is a distinct absence of 5α-reductase activity, which converts T to DHT, while androgen receptor levels are normal (Walsh et al., 1974).

TABLE 4

Proposed Classification of the Androgen Resistance Syndromes on the Basis of Anatomic, Genetic, and Hormonal Characteristics [Madden et al., 1975]

		Phenotype					Endocrine profile relative to normal male			
Disorder	Inheritance	Müllerian ducts	Wolffian ducts	Urogenital sinus	Urogenital tubercle, swelling, and folds	Breast	Testosterone production	Estrogen production	LH	FSH
Complete testicular feminization	X-linked recessive	Not detectable	Not detectable	Female	Female	Female	High	High	High	Normal
Incomplete testicular feminization	?	Not detectable	Male	Female	Partial labioscrotal fusion and clitoromegaly	Female	High	High	High	High
Familial incomplete male pseudohermaphroditism, Type 1	Probable X-linked recessive	Not detectable	Variable from male to incomplete development	Variable from male to female	Incomplete male development	Female	High	High	High	Normal
Familial incomplete male pseudohermaphroditism, Type 2	Autosomal recessive	Not detectable	Male	Female	Clitoromegaly	Male	Normal	Normal	Normal	Normal

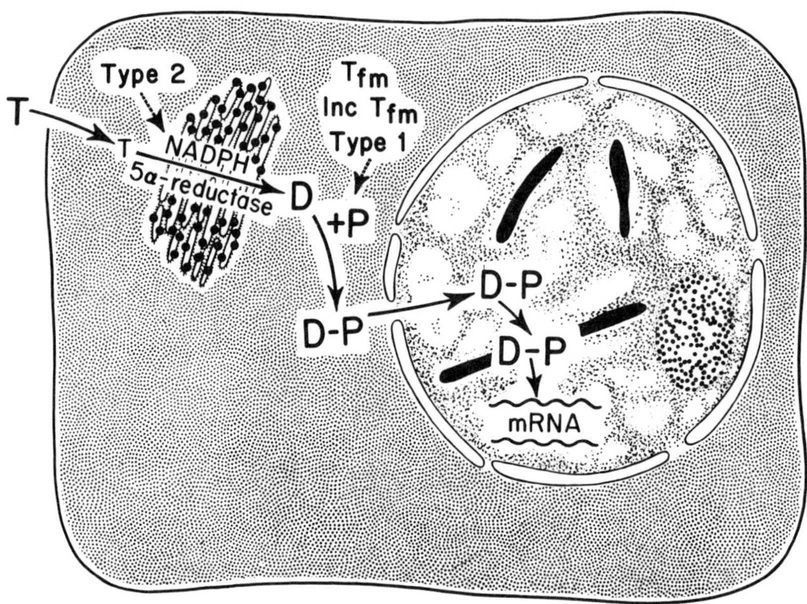

Figure 14. Schematic representation of the mechanism of action of testosterone. D = dihydrotestosterone; Inc Tfm = incomplete testicular feminization; mRNA = messenger RNA; P = androgen receptor protein; T = testosterone; Tfm = testicular feminization; Type 1 = Reifenstein syndrome; Type 2 = steroid 5α-reductase deficiency. [Wilson]

Wilson suggests the possibility that, normally, androgens like DHT may act synergistically with estrogens in external genitalia to cause differentiation, whereas the differentiation of internal reproduction tract structures may require only androgens such as T. This suggestion is based on evidence that estradiol and androstanediol act synergistically to promote growth of adult structures such as the prostate (Walsh and Wilson, 1976).

Wilson thinks that the first three mutations described in Table 4 influence the androgen receptor protein (Griffin et al., 1976). Employing whole-cell binding and subcellular fractionation techniques with fibroblasts cultured from these patients, Wilson and colleagues noted a profound deficiency in DHT binding. In cytosol from the normal patient's fibroblasts, a 4S- and 8S-binding component was observed, while both of these are apparently absent or at very low levels in these individuals. Yet, as noted above, Type 2 pseudohermaphrodites are normal in this regard, indicating that pseudohermaphroditism per se does not affect this parameter. Wilson does not know the nature of these mutations. One possibility is that they are regulatory, affecting synthesis rates of receptors. Or the mutations may be allelic, such as in hemoglobins S and C, or they could involve individual subunits of the active receptor protein.

We do know a little bit more about the *Tfm* mutation in the mouse. As shown by a number of workers, the 8S-binding protein is apparently absent in the *Tfm* male, whereas the carrier female is intermediate between the *Tfm* male and the normal female. In addition, in the submandibular gland there exists a 2.6S protein in all four genotypes, but its relationship to the receptor is unclear. If the partially purified 8S receptor, isolated at low ionic strength, is recentrifuged in the presence of 0.4 M KC1, it dissociates into smaller components that are similar to the 2.6S protein. These observations are consistent with the possibility that in the *Tfm* mouse the steroid receptor complex does not activate and, thereby, does not gain entry into the cell nucleus.

Going beyond 5α-reductase and androgen receptors, Wilson has some interesting new information on two rather well-studied patients. These genetic males appear phenotypically almost like *Tfm,* except they do not feminize at puberty. However, they possess apparently normal 5α-reductase levels, as well as 8S receptor protein; yet they seem to be completely resistant to their own androgens. Wilson has hypothesized that they possess a mutation(s) at the nuclear acceptor site or at some more distal point in the sequelae of androgen action.

It is interesting to note that there are more mutations for androgen action than for all other steroids put together. There is no convincing evidence for hereditary resistance to estrogen action or hereditary defects in estrogen synthesis, nor have naturally occurring mutations involving aldosterone or corticosterone resistance due to receptor abnormality been characterized. There are two possible explanations for this: First, since the mutation affecting the DHT-binding protein is X-linked, the disorder is expressed more often in genetic males due to its single X chromosome; whereas, if the genes regulating the other binding proteins are located on autosomes, absence of the binding protein would only be expressed in the homozygous state. This could explain part of the discrepancy. Second, another possibility is that steroid hormones other than androgens are essential for life. Estradiol is probably essential for implantation, and aldosterone and glucocorticoids are also essential. Therefore, a mutation affecting the normal action of these hormones would be lethal at some phase or other of embryogenesis.

Morphological Sex Differences in Mammalian Brain and Their Possible Origins

A popular working hypothesis is that differences in circuitry of the brain underlie sex differences in behavior and physiology. Given this hypothesis, there are a number of ways in which a suspected sexually dimorphic brain area could manifest these differences. These are: (1) Afferent pattern–neurons could actually be connected with different impinging inputs or there could be differences in the relative weighting of the same set of inputs. (2) Within structure–differences in the way information is processed or routed through. (3) Efferent pattern–differences in projections from the region in question. These potential differences require different techniques for their detection: (1) or (2) might be detected by using Golgi techniques; whereas (3) would require transport, degeneration, and electrophysiological techniques.

Several studies have suggested possible structural dimorphisms of this kind. In electrophysiological studies, Dyer and colleagues (1976) stimulated the corticomedial amygdala and recorded from the preoptic area (POA) and anterior hypothalamic area (AHA). Many more of the POA-AHA cells that projected to the medial basal hypothalamus were driven by amygdala stimulation in males and TP-treated females than in females or in neonatally castrated males, suggesting a functional "wiring" difference that is under neonatal hormonal control. Earlier studies by Pfaff (1966) and especially Dörner and Staudt (e.g., 1968) demonstrated a sexual dimorphism in cell nuclear size in various hypothalamic regions that was regulated by neonatal hormonal conditions. These differences may indicate dimorphism in "within structure" processing of information but might also reflect sex differences in afferent or efferent connections. Staudt and Dörner (1976) also found a sexual dimorphism in cell nuclear size in the central and medial amygdala regions that is under the neonatal influence of sex hormones.

The now classic morphological study (Figure 15) suggesting "wiring diagram" sex differences in the brain is the electron microscope analysis of Raisman and Field (1971, 1973) in which they found, in the bed nucleus of the stria terminalis, more nonstrial-derived spine synapses in females and neonatally castrated males than in males or neonatally testosterone-treated females. Raisman and Field found no differences in the termination pattern of amygdaloid stria terminalis afferents, in contrast to the study of Dyer and co-workers (1976) from which one would have predicted a difference in strial-derived synapses. Raisman and Field have carried out further descriptive Golgi and quantitative electron microscope analyses of hypothalamic regions that have revealed no other dimorphisms in other strial terminations or nonstrial synaptic patterns.

Stimulated by numerous suggestions of functional sexual dimorphism in the preoptic area and by the Raisman and Field work, Carter and Greenough (see Greenough et al., 1977a) have begun to examine the cellular basis of these differences. They studied golden hamsters because of the minimal dimorphism in body weight and, as they found, in brain dimensions. In addition, male sexual behavior in the hamster is markedly sexually dimorphic (Carter et al., 1972).

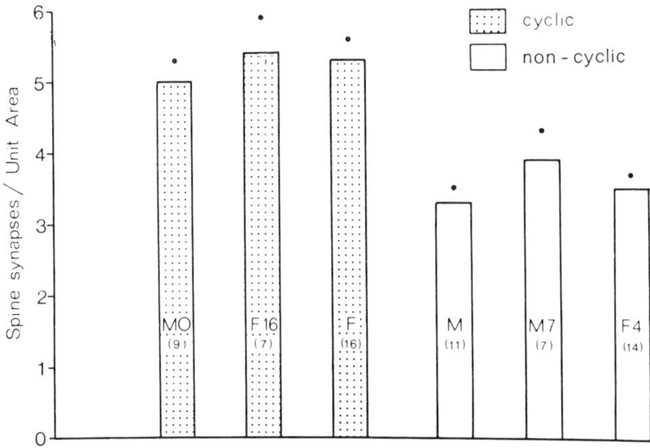

Figure 15. A bar diagram showing the mean incidences (dot, one standard error) of nonstrial synapses per grid square in the POA in each of the 6 groups of animals (cyclic groups shaded). The number of brackets is the number of animals in each group: M = normal males, M0 = males castrated at birth, M7 = males castrated at 7 days of age, F = normal females, F4 = females given 1.25 mg of TP on day 4, F16 = females similarly treated on day 16. [Raisman and Field, 1973]

Dorsomedial POA in Golgi-stained hamster brain revealed the same basic types of neurons described by Field and Sherlock (1975) in the rat. Camera lucida drawings of these neurons were initially analyzed for sex differences in: (1) length of dendrites, (2) number of dendrites, (3) number of bifurcations, (4) number of branches of various orders, and (5) estimates of the total amount of dendrite of a cell using a concentric circle grid. In the past, procedures (1) to (5) had shown effects of early environmental experiences on cortical neuron morphology (e.g., Greenough, 1975). Measures (1) to (4) produced no clear sex differences applied to each or to all of the three basic cell types. Procedure (5) indicated that neurons in males had about 5% more "total dendrite" than those in females.

Results from the last technique also hinted that male and female dendrites might actually be concentrated in different regions within the dorsomedial POA. To measure this, Greenough and coworkers (1977b) employed a grid network and scored the number of dendritic crossings on an X-Y plane, using known neuroanatomical structures as landmarks (Figure 16). The results of this analysis indicated that the density of dendrites in the male was slightly higher than in the female in a circumscribed region of the dorsomedial POA, ventral to the anterior commissure. This effect can also be visualized graphically (Figure 17): the female dendritic density dips in this region and the male peaks. The effects of neonatal hormonal manipulations on these patterns were not clear cut, although TP-treated females did become more malelike and castrated males did become more femalelike.

These studies involved animals that were gonadectomized at 80 days of age and then treated identically with exogenous hormones until 235 days of age to test adult behavioral sensitivity to hormones. The POA differences were therefore not due to activational effects of different sex hormones in adulthood. Moreover, in normal intact animals, sexual dimorphism was still noted in the same area (Greenough et al., 1977b). Greenough and Carter conclude that there is a dimorphism in hamster dorsomedial POA. The male has neurons that tend to send dendrites to the center of that structure, whereas neurons in the female do not. This phenomenon is only partially influenced by neonatal hormonal manipulation.

Greenough and collaborators (1977b) have also studied the suprachiasmatic nucleus (SCN). The SCN was defined as a rectilinear

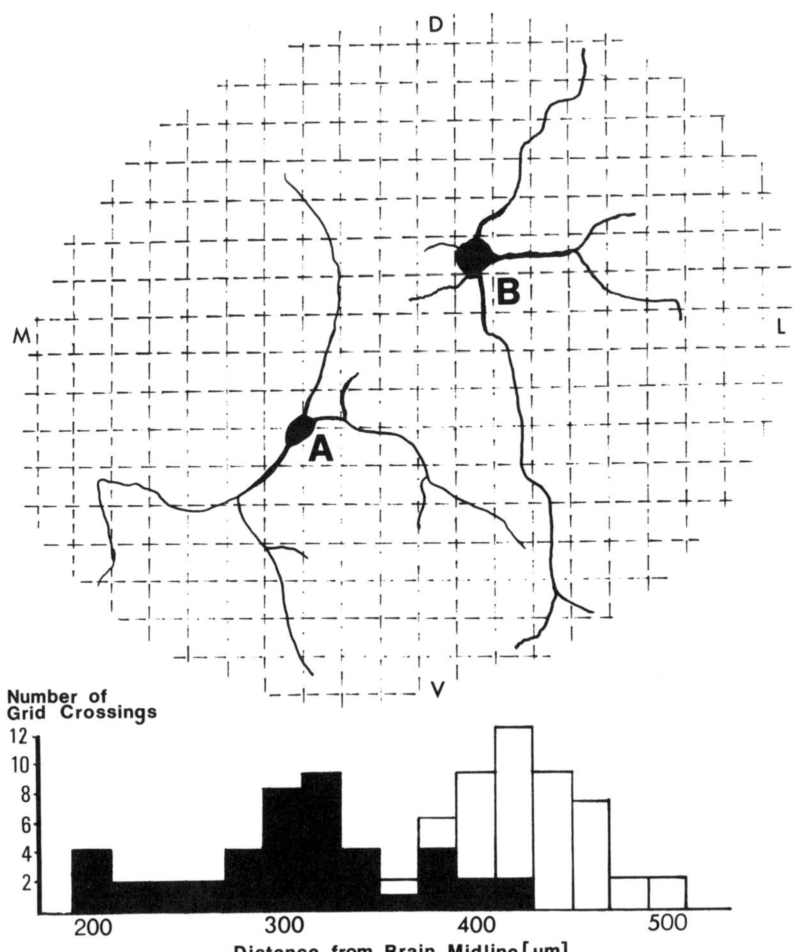

Figure 16. Schematic representation of the scoring method used to quantify dendrite density distribution. Hatched lines illustrate a transparent overlay used to score dendritic branching. Each square is a 20-μm equivalent. Solid bars represent total dendritic grid crossings from neuron A. Open bars represent total crossings from neuron B. Adding grid coordinates to cell body location coordinates (distance from anatomical landmarks) for all neurons and averaging yields the histograms in Figure 17. Summing across only the anterior-posterior dimension yields a two-dimensional relative density plot as in Figure 18. D = dorsal; L = lateral; M = medial; V = ventral. [Greenough et al., 1977b]

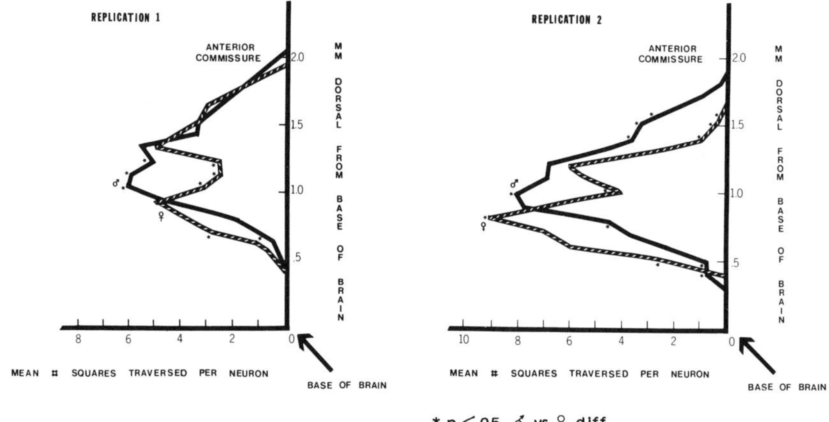

Figure 17. Average number of 20-μm squares intersected at indicated depths in the POA by dendrites of neurons sampled from the dorsomedial POA. Arrows to left indicate depth of cell body sample region. Significant differences between males (solid line) and females (striped line) are indicated by *. [Greenough et al., 1977b]

solid centered over the optic chiasm, 250 μ high, 600 μ wide, and extending 1000 μ posterior to the anterior crossing of the optic chiasm; this region is only approximately congruent with the SCN seen in Nissl-stained sections. It has been suggested that the SCN interacts with or drives the POA cyclically to produce the LH surge necessary for female ovulation, not present in males (Rusak and Zucker, 1975; Stetson and Watson-Whitmyre, 1976). Again using the grid-based reconstruction technique, Greenough and collaborators observed a central concentration of dendrites in males and a more peripherally distributed concentration of SCN neuron dendrites in females (Figure 18).

How do these dimorphisms arise? Greenough presented four possibilities:

1. *Differential growth rates.* If hormones or other mediators of sexual dimorphism slowed or increased neuronal process growth rate, they might make contact with afferents growing through the area at different times.

2. *Triggered formation of connections.* Hormones might cause (or prevent) synaptic contacts to form between selected neuronal populations whose processes were proximate during development.

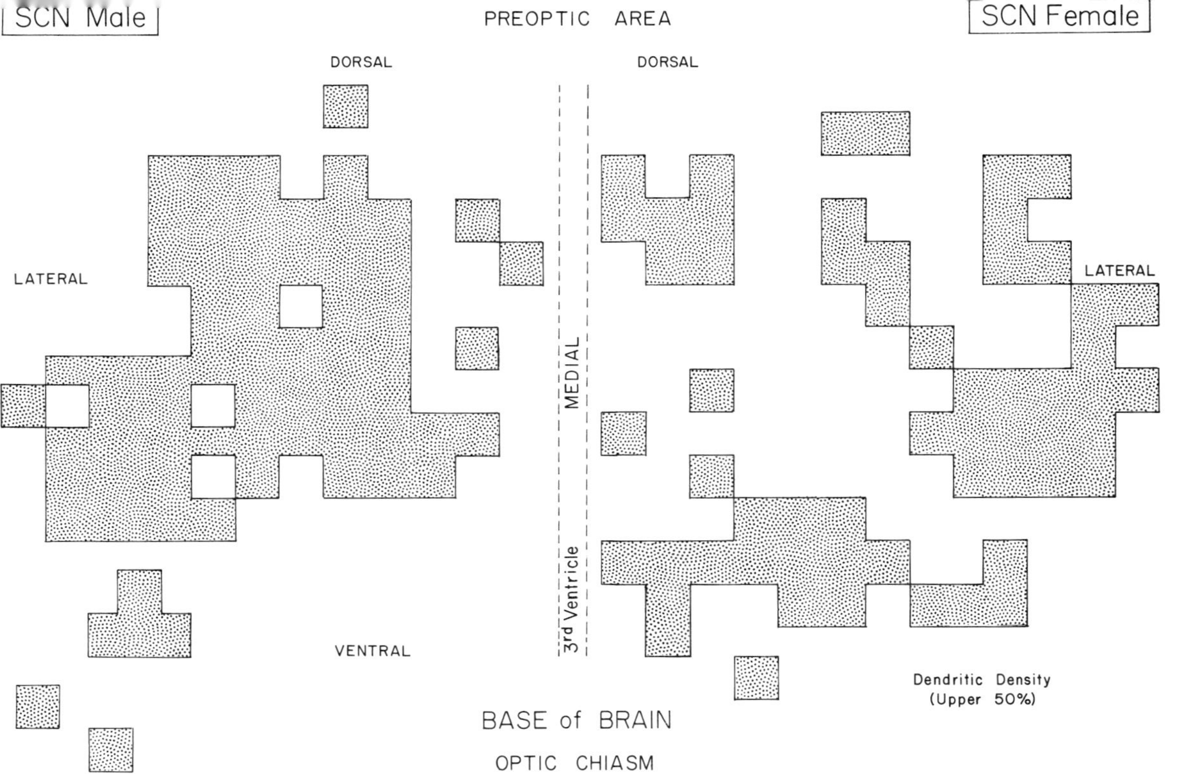

Figure 18. Relative density of dendrites from SCN neurons in 40 sq. μm divisions of SCN. Shaded areas have greater than the median frequency of dendrites. Males, projected as if the left SCN, have a concentration of dendrites in the center; females, projected as if in the right SCN, show distributed density. Note nondimorphic ventrolateral concentration in both sexes. [Greenough]

3. *Directed growth.* Hormones might alter chemoaffinity patterns, resulting in differentially directed growth patterns (paralleling findings of retinotectal connection research).

4. *Selective preservation.* Initial growth may be uniform across sexes with hormones "stamping in" some connections, while the remainder deteriorate or while others are selected in the absence of hormones.

Current data do not allow us to choose from these alternatives. However, we can see dimorphism in the dendritic pattern of adult neurons in accord with the dimorphism in overall dendritic pattern of a brain region. Neurons of SCN were grouped according to the quadrant (e.g., dorsomedial, ventrolateral) of SCN containing their cell bodies. The terminations of dendrites were counted in each equal octant around the cell body and are represented in Figure 19 as lines, connected by shading, extending from a central cell body location. Neurons in all quadrants in males extend dendrites toward the center of the structure, in accord with the SCN central density in Figure 18, while

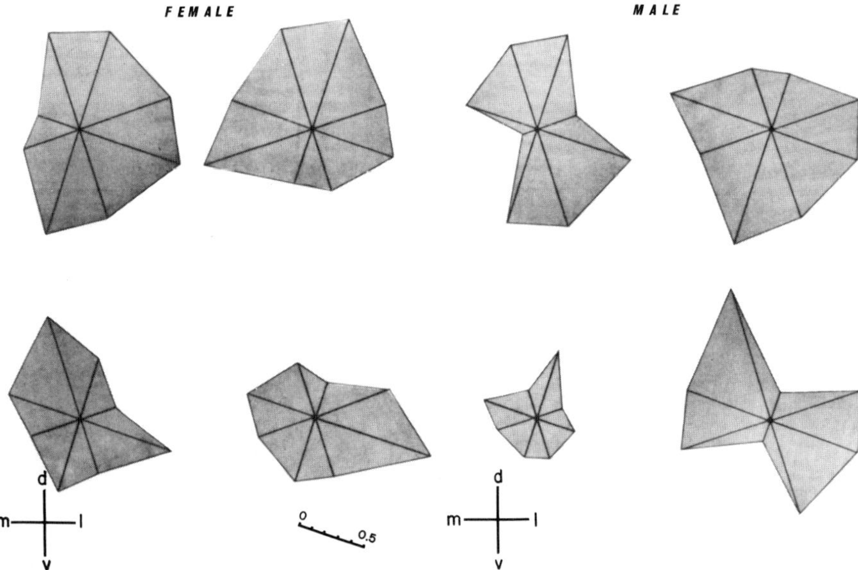

Figure 19. Lengths of lines represent number of dendritic branches terminating in each octant around the cell body in SCN neurons. Neurons in each quadrant of SCN are grouped for analysis. Both males and females projected as if in the right SCN. [Greenough]

neurons in females avoid the center, as suggested by the reduced central density in Figure 18. Developmental studies should shed light on the process whereby this dimorphism at the individual neuronal level is achieved.

Sexual Dimorphism in the Size of Rat Medial Preoptic Nucleus

Gorski admitted that prior to the Raisman and Field (1973) study the existence of a morphological basis for sexual differentiation seemed to him very unlikely. His general conception was that steroids altered responsivity of the system, not its morphology. In support of this notion, one finds for example that, by testing rats under the appropriate conditions, it is possible to induce female patterns of sexual behavior in males (Davidson, 1969). Although the male rat has the capacity to exhibit female sexual behavior, it is more difficult to activate this system in males than in females. However, the original work of Raisman and Field (1973) and then the studies of Greenough and colleagues (1977) and Nottebohm and Arnold (1976) convinced Gorski and Christensen to reexamine morphological characteristics in the rat brain. Their subsequent finding of a morphological sex difference relates to a limited portion of the medial preoptic nucleus in the preoptic-anterior hypothalamic region of the brain (Gorski et al., 1977, 1978). Adult Sprague-Dawley rats were gonadectomized 2 weeks before sacrifice and brain removal, and thick frozen sections (60 μ) were cut and stained with either thionine or cresyl violet. Gorski found a marked sex difference in a densely staining portion of the medial preoptic nucleus. It is important to remember that this is just a component of the larger medial preoptic area.

The size of this densely staining area was found to be larger in males than in females. This difference is so striking that one can readily discriminate male versus female solely by visual examination of slides that include this brain area. To obtain some quantitative information so that he could study the influence of hormones both in adults and prenatally, Gorski utilized the following procedure to measure the volume and location of this more densely staining area. Three individuals, independently and without knowledge of treatment, each outlined the densely stained nucleus; then Gorski superimposed these outlines, also without knowledge of treatment. He next measured the weight of tracing vellum contained within the visual average of the three outlines to calculate the nucleus volume. This method of ascertaining the size of the sexually dimorphic area had an element of subjectivity; but at least it was unbiased as to treatment as far as he could determine.

Measurements of this nucleus in six males and females indicated its center anterior to the suprachiasmatic nucleus by an average of 0.65 mm for the males and 0.58 mm for the females. In addition, the nucleus center was posterior to the anterior commissure by 0.40 mm for males and 0.26 mm for females and lateral to the midline by 0.37 mm for males and 0.12 mm for females (Figure 20).

The major sex difference was in the volume of this nucleus, which was estimated to be 0.96 ± 0.06 mm^3 in the male and 0.12 ± 0.03 mm^3 in the female. The volume of darkly staining cells that Gorski refers to as the medial preoptic nucleus had a volume 8 times greater in males than in females. Aside from body weight, which was greater in males than in females, other parameters were not significantly different. These included size and weight of the brain, height of the

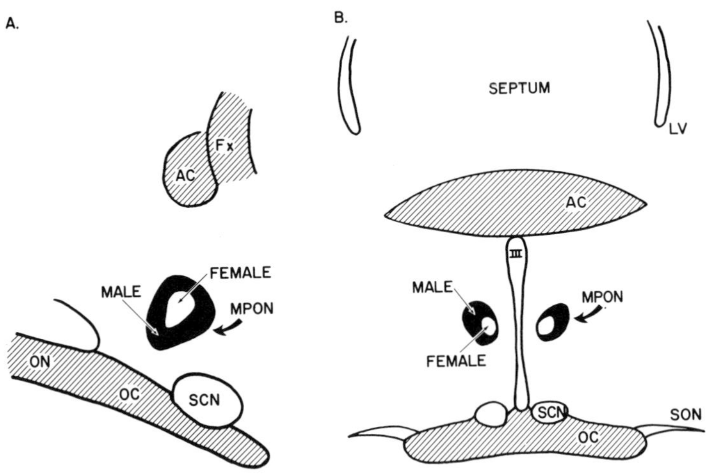

Figure 20. Schematic localization of the sexually dimorphic component of the medial preoptic nucleus (MPON) in the sagittal (A) and coronal (B) planes. As shown, this region in the female can be completely contained in that of the male. AC = anterior commissure; Fx = fornix; LV = lateral ventricle; OC = optic chiasm; ON = optic nerve; SCN = suprachiasmatic nucleus; SON = supraoptic nucleus; III = third ventricle. [Gorski et al., 1978]

preoptic area from the anterior commissure to the optic chiasm, width from midline to the lateral border of the optic chiasm, and width of the septum.

One question is whether this gross sexual dimorphism is dependent on adult hormones. To study this, Gorski started with adult gonadectomized rats and gave either hormone replacement or other treatments (Gorski et al., 1978). One group received a regimen of female hormones, estrogen and progesterone, which normally restores lordosis in the female. Another group of males and females was given testosterone at a dose that would normally restore male sexual behavior. In others, thyroid function was attenuated by treating the animals with propylthiouracil, a goitrogen, and the weight of the thyroids in these animals was almost 6 times the weight of the thyroids in the control animals. They also dehydrated some animals. The reason for this was to rule out the possibility that this sexually dimorphic area is related to the nucleus circularis, which Hatton (1976) has regarded as an osmoreceptor. The nucleus circularis is, however, located more caudally. Finally, he adrenalectomized a group of animals, but 2 weeks after adrenalectomy he found levels of corticoids that were more or less normal. Apparently there is enough accessory adrenal tissue in this strain of rats that they were not adrenalectomized physiologically, and Gorski did not analyze the brain data of these animals.

The results of these treatments confirmed the highly significant sex difference in volume of this nucleus, but there was no significant treatment effect (Figure 21). This sex difference did appear specific; again, other than body weight, no significant differences were noted in terms of brain weight or in terms of preoptic height or width or in septal height. In terms of nuclei, it is impractical to measure all of those in the brain, but the suprachiasmatic nucleus that was analyzed did not show these large sex differences. Statistical analysis did suggest a possible sex difference in volume of the suprachiasmatic nucleus (Figure 22). It should be remembered that Gorski's procedures are not that precise; when he repeated eight different measurements, he found an average variance in his measures of approximately 15%. Although he cannot discount the possibility that there are other sexual dimorphisms in the rat brain, the differences he found in the rat suprachiasmatic nucleus are not sufficiently great, given the variability of the measurements, to convince one that this is a real sex difference.

Another very important question is whether or not the observed sex difference in volume of the intensely staining component of

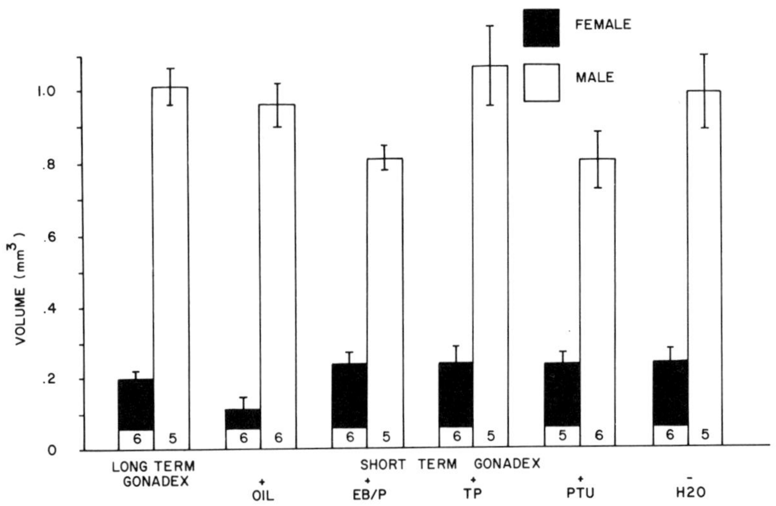

Figure 21. Evidence that the sex difference in mean volume (± standard error) of the intensely staining component of the medial preoptic area is independent of the following hormone regimes in the adult: EB/P = estradiol benzoate/progesterone; TP = testosterone propionate; PTU = propylthiouracil; $-H_2O$ = water deprivation. The numbers at the base of each bar indicate the number of brains analyzed. [Gorski et al., 1978]

the medial preoptic nucleus is sexually differentiated. To date the studies of Gorski and co-workers (1978) indicate that it is. They compared brains of adult males and females given various neonatal treatments. Control females received oil treatment neonatally while two other groups of females received either 90 μg or 1 mg of testosterone propionate in a similar injection on day 4 of life. One group of males was castrated on day 1 under hypothermia anesthesia. Gorski (1967) calls these FALES, meaning feminine males. The control group of males received a sham operation also under hypothermia anesthesia on the first day of life.

Statistical analysis of the data on suprachiasmatic nuclear volume showed no significant difference for that nucleus (Figure 23). However, the medial preoptic nuclear volume in the control male was significantly greater than for any of the other groups. In addition, this region of the neonatally castrated males (FALE) and of the females treated with 1 mg of testosterone propionate were both significantly greater in volume than that of the control females. It is interesting to

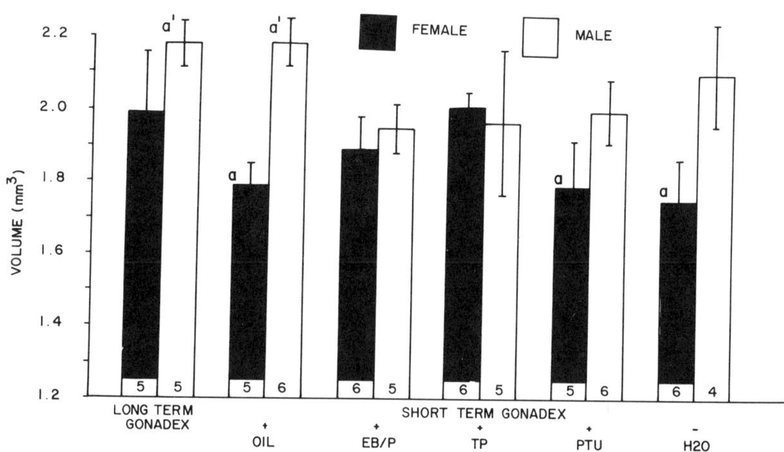

Figure 22. The influence of hormone treatment of the adult gonadectomized rat on the volume of the suprachiasmatic nucleus. See Figure 21 for further details. a′ significantly ($P<0.05$) larger than a. [Gorski et al., 1978]

note that nuclear volume in the neonatally castrated male is not the same as that of the female, nor is the nucleus of the androgenized female the size found in the control male. This suggests that there may be either prenatal hormonal influences on the volume of this nucleus, or a genetic component, or both.

An important but still unanswered question relates to the first appearance of this dimorphism. Very preliminary data suggest that at 22 days pc the male and female are equal (both large), and that the sexual dimorphism begins to appear within a few days after birth. The fact that the above volume measurements were obtained by analysis of thick sections has prevented Gorski from performing a differential cell count within this region. However, he has now determined that the sexual dimorphism is also detectable in paraffin sections cut at 10 μm, but the dimorphism is clearly less marked. Although a total cell count (neurons and glia) within a narrow strip across the nuclear region has established the existence of the medial preoptic nucleus on a quantitative basis, these preliminary data have not provided a statistically significant quantitative expression of the obvious sexual dimorphism. Gorski is now in the process of expanding both the size of the window of analysis and the classifications of cell types counted. Although the

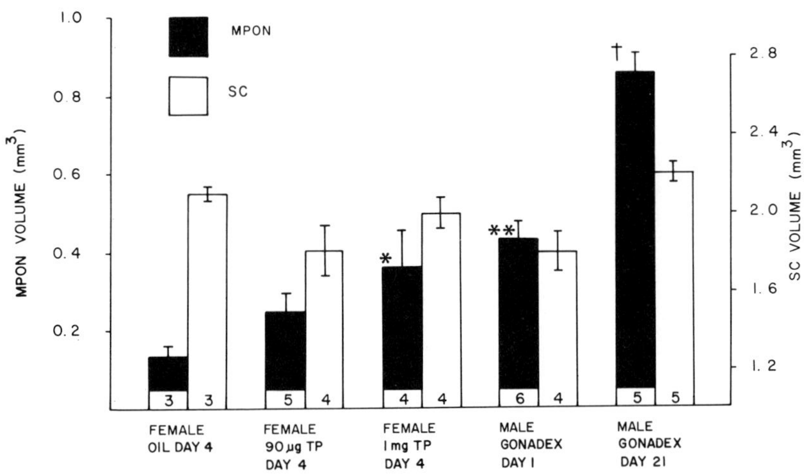

Figure 23. Evidence that the sex difference in mean volume (± standard error) of the intensely staining component of the medial preoptic nucleus (MPON) is dependent upon neonatal hormone treatment. The volume of the suprachiasmatic nucleus (SC) is also shown. Females were given oil, 90 μg, or 1 mg of testosterone propionate (TP) on day 4 of life, and ovariectomized 2 weeks before sacrifice. Males were castrated either on day 1 or 21. † = significantly ($P<0.05$) larger than any other group; ** = significantly ($P<0.01$) larger than oil-treated female; * = significantly ($P<0.05$) larger than oil-treated female. [Gorski et al., 1978]

sexual dimorphism appears clearly to reside in neurons, questions of cell size, density, and staining intensity remain to be answered.

Gorski presently has no idea what specific function, if any, this area might have. Nuclear volume per se is not consistent with the pattern of gonadotropin regulation exhibited by the animals; i.e., the female and FALE will exhibit the cyclic pattern of gonadotropin release, but the testosterone-treated female rats and control males will not. A similar lack of correlation exists between nuclear volume and the ability to display lordosis behavior; i.e., high levels of female sexual behavior can readily be elicited from control females and FALES but not from testosterone-treated females or males. (Compare these observations with nuclear volumes shown in Figure 23.) One parameter that might relate to the morphological difference is male sexual behavior, but Gorski lacks sufficient data to make a conclusion in this regard. Other studies initiated before these findings have shown that lesions (Christensen et al., 1977) or hormonal implants (Christensen and Gorski, 1978) around this area can influence male sexual activity, but these interventions were not aimed specifically at this nucleus and are just suggestive. Gerall* has additional evidence that very discrete lesions are most effective in disrupting male rat sexual behavior when placed in the area of this nucleus, rather than in the midline structures at the base of the ventricle as one might expect.

Whether a similar sex difference within the medial preoptic nucleus exists in other species is uncertain. Greenough and Carter's analysis (see above) in the hamster involved an area of the preoptic primarily dorsal to the portion of the POA in question. From simple histological analysis of sections taken from the preoptic area of four mouse brains, Gorski was unable to determine which was male or female. Thus, a sex difference, if it exists in the mouse, is not the obvious and dramatic difference seen in Sprague-Dawley rats.

The obviousness of this observed sex difference in the rat might make it an excellent model to study by various histological and biochemical techniques in order to determine possible connections and functions in reference to other brain areas. The punch technique to isolate and analyze biochemically small tissue areas and nuclei indicates a high level of aromatase in this area and high levels of testosterone conversion to estrogens. Autoradiographic results of testosterone are not conclusive because of its ready conversion in neural tissue. There is evidence for estrogen receptors in this area, but it is not a region of maximal density for such receptors. The question of androgen receptors will have to await the publication of dihydrotestosterone autoradiograms. Transmitters in this area should also be looked at, but this question is complicated by the fact that the area is rich in both terminations from other regions and cell bodies that have endings in other areas.

Sex Differences in Avian Brain Structure and Their Possible Origins

As noted above by Nottebohm, sexually dimorphic vocal behavior occurs in many oscine songbirds: while males sing elaborate songs learned by reference to auditory information, females do not sing or sing considerably less. In the European chaffinch, occurrence of song

*Unpublished observations.

depends on the presence of testosterone (Collard and Grevendal, 1946; Poulsen, 1951; Thorpe, 1958; Nottebohm, 1969). Female chaffinches can be induced to sing following testosterone propionate treatment and under those conditions are capable of imitating male song (Hooker, 1968). In the Australian zebra finch, male song develops after early castration, but testosterone is necessary for the high rates of singing typical of intact adult males (Pröve, 1974; Arnold, 1975a,b). In canaries early castration interferes with the development of loud stable song in first-year males.* However, whereas female canaries respond to androgen treatment with malelike song (Leonard, 1939; Shoemaker, 1939; Baldwin et al., 1940; Herrick and Harris, 1957), female zebra finches seem to lack this ability (Arnold, 1974).

Recent work has shown that canary song, and presumably that of other songbirds, is controlled by a discrete set of brain areas: the hyperstriatum ventrale, pars caudale (HVc), area X of lobus parolfactorius, the robust nucleus of the archistriatum (RA), and the caudal half of the hypoglossal nucleus (nXIIts). Motoneurons in the latter structure innervate the syringeal musculature and are thus responsible for the patterning of song (Nottebohm et al., 1976). HVc, area X, and RA are telencephalic structures. A fifth area, nucleus magnocellularis anterior of the neostriatum, innervates both HVc and RA (Figure 24).† All five brain areas are markedly larger in male than in female canaries. An even more marked sexual dimorphism in brain structure is present in zebra finches (Figure 25). In this case the Nissl and fiber stains used failed to reveal a female area X (Nottebohm and Arnold, 1976). The more marked sexual dimorphism of the zebra finch brain may relate to the fact that adult female zebra finches cannot be brought into song even under the influence of testosterone (Arnold, 1974). Of course, a dimorphism such as that observed in the adult songbird brain may result from various influences such as genetic factors, early hormonal influences on brain differentiation, the effects of use and disuse, the effects of learning, and the direct effect of the hormones themselves on the tissue of the adult brain.

Intact adult female canaries implanted with a pellet of TP come into malelike song, though they tend to produce many fewer note types. In such females studied by Nottebohm (1979), 1 month after

*F. Nottebohm, unpublished observations.

†F. Nottebohm and D.B. Kelley, manuscript in preparation.

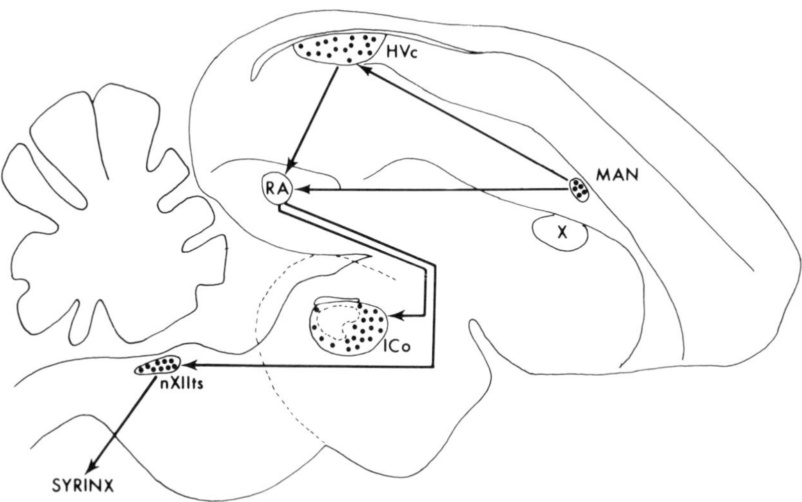

Figure 24. Schematic sagittal section of the canary brain on which brain structures and pathways implicated in song control have been outlined. Unilateral lesions restricted to hyperstriatum ventrale, pars caudale (HVc) result in major song disruptions. Degenerating fibers traced from such lesions end in area X (pathway not shown) and nucleus robustus archistriatalis (RA). Unilateral lesions of RA also disrupt song. A direct pathway links RA to nXIIts, the motor nucleus innervating the syrinx. Nucleus intercollicularis of the midbrain (ICo) also receives a projection from RA. Nucleus magnocellularis anterior of the neostriatum (MAN) projects both to HVc and RA (Nottebohm et al., 1976). Solid dots indicate the presence of labeled cells after systemic injection of tritiated testosterone in male zebra finches, in which vocal control pathways are similar to those described for the canary. [Arnold et al., 1976]

onset of testosterone treatment HVc and RA are 60 to 65% larger than in control females (Figure 26). Hence, at least half of the gross difference in volume of male and female HVc and RA can be attributed to hormonal effects in the adult brain. The finding that hormone treatment could have such a marked effect in the brain of adult and sexually mature individuals was so unexpected that these experiments have been repeated under better-controlled conditions. Male and female canaries were gonadectomized 1 to 3 weeks after hatching. At 11 months of age half of the females (n = 5) were treated for 1 month with cholesterol, the other half (n = 5) with testosterone. Only the T-treated females developed malelike song. In the latter, HVc was 90% larger than that of cholesterol-treated controls, and RA was 53% larger. The early castrated males (n = 10) also were sacrificed at 1 year of age. Their HVc was

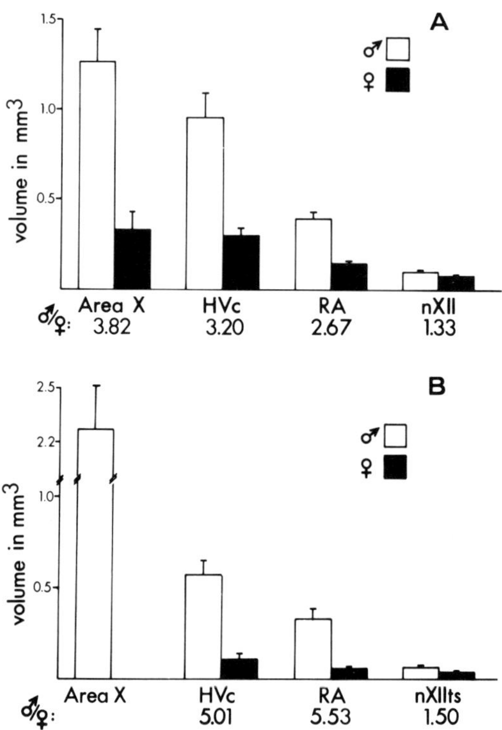

Figure 25. Volumes occupied by four neural regions associated with vocal behavior in males and their corresponding volumes in females. A. Illustration of observations in canaries. B. Illustration of observations in zebra finches. Each bar represents the mean of the total (right plus left) volumes of each area sampled, and the vertical line above the bar is the standard deviation of the individual values. The ratio of the male to the female mean is given for each region. [Nottebohm and Arnold, 1976]

30% smaller than that of intact siblings (n = 10), whereas RA was 35% smaller. Two males, castrated as year-old adults and which failed to sing during the following year, also had markedly smaller HVc and RA than 2-year-old intact controls (n = 5) (Nottebohm, 1979).

At this point the vocal control system of the songbird brain looms as very attractive material to study the ontogeny of sexually dimorphic brain pathways: the areas involved develop late in ontogeny,* at least some areas concentrate testosterone or its metabolites (Arnold

*F. Nottebohm, unpublished observations.

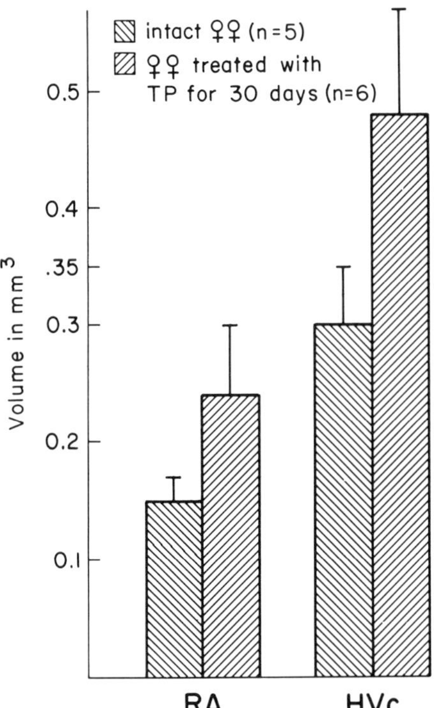

Figure 26. Effects of testosterone treatment on *adult* female canaries during 1 month. These birds received a 10-mg subcutaneous pellet of testosterone propionate. Note that both HVc and RA show a significant increase in volume. The TP-treated females developed malelike song. [Nottebohm]

et al., 1976; Figure 26), and their connectivity and behavioral role have been well demonstrated. Future developments should render this system even more interesting.

Neurite Outgrowth in Cultured Mouse Hypothalamus: A Possible Model System?

Morphological sex differences in the adult brain are the final result of the sexual differentiation process and do not indicate what cellular events actually produced them. Toran-Allerand's studies are directed toward describing responses of relatively undifferentiated CNS tissue to gonadal steroids, estradiol and testosterone, using an organotypic tissue culture system. The organotypic culture system is so named because it allows fragments of fetal or neonatal brain tissue to survive and differentiate in a manner comparable to that found in vivo. It is based on the premise that cellular interactions among the cells of a brain region and the three-dimensional architectonics of the interacting cells are fundamental to the developmental process. By attempting to preserve as many neuronal and nonneuronal cell types as possible, one avoids introducing the unavoidable bias of selection inherent in dissociated cell culture methods.

Organotypic cultures differentiate extensively and exhibit remarkable morphological fidelity with comparably aged brain structures by both light and electron microscopy. In addition, the de novo formation of synapses, myelin sheaths, and releasing hormones in culture suggest that there is a preservation of many of the intrinsic characteristics of nerve tissue. In Toran-Allerand's experiments, six coronal sections, 300 μm thick, are prepared from newborn mouse brain and divided at the third ventricle into homologous or mirror pairs. One of each pair may be subjected to experimental manipulation, e.g., hormone treatment, and the other half serves as control. Toran-Allerand observes the rate of outgrowth and morphology of neurites, a general term for presumptive axons and dendrites. The culture technique is that of Maximow with a nutrient medium containing amino acids, vitamins, glucose, and horse serum, and no antibiotics. Steroids are added by dissolving them in saline or by adsorbing them to 0.5% bovine serum albumin.

Regardless of the genetic sex of the culture, addition of estradiol or testosterone from time of explantation enhances the outgrowth of neurites from the preoptic area and from the infundibular and premamillary levels of the hypothalamus. Other regions grow but show no effect of added steriod. Toran-Allerand is still not able to indicate the exact nuclei from which this growth occurs. The steroid effect is not seen if the meninges are present at explantation. A remarkable feature of the outgrowth stimulated by gonadal steroids is that it is so persistent, compared to control pairs where outgrowth tends to be short-lived in the absence of a target (i.e., other neural tissue) with neurites turning around and growing back into the explant. Yet the stimulated outgrowth appears to be largely an exaggeration of the normal pattern seen in control cultures.

Relatively few neurites seem to contribute to plexuses, suggesting that outgrowth involves formation of new branches and that the steroid effect is limited to a subpopulation of neurons in the culture. This is in keeping with the in vivo distribution of gonadal steroid-concentrating neurons, which are discretely localized within the preoptic area and hypothalamus. Recent autoradiographic studies on Toran-Allerand's cultures by Gerlach and McEwen (Toran-Allerand et al., 1978) reveal small clusters of ^{3}H-estradiol-concentrating neurons in the preoptic area and in the infundibular level of the hypothalamus, both steroid-responsive areas in culture, but not in the anterior hypothalamus, a nonresponsive area in culture. The neuronal specificity of the effect is further supported by the observation of single neurons contributing heavily to the outgrowth through extensive branching of neurites.

Because Toran-Allerand uses horse serum, which contains some estrogen, it was necessary for her to try to remove this estrogen from serum and observe the consequences for growth of control cultures. This was accomplished either by using antibodies against estradiol or by treating horse serum with charcoal or Sephadex LH-20. What happened was exactly the opposite of adding steroid to cultures. Compared to control cultures, paired halves treated with antibodies or with serum treated with charcoal or LH-20 showed less neurite outgrowth and gave indications of having larger numbers of neuroblasts with little process formation (Figure 27).

Toran-Allerand added various steroids to cultures (Figure 27). Testosterone alone produced minimal neurite outgrowth, whereas another androgen, 5α-dihydrotestosterone, in similar concentrations to T or 17β-estradiol (E_2) produced no effect whatsoever. These results are consistent with the notion that T acts to produce brain sexual differentiation in the mouse and rat via its conversion to estradiol (see later discussion of this idea). In further support of a specific estrogen effect, Toran-Allerand observed that a nonsteroidal antiestrogen, CI-628, inhibits neurite outgrowth produced by estrogens present in the horse serum by at least 50%. This observation suggests the possible involvement of intracellular estrogen receptors, the presence of which in the culture is indicated by the Gerlach-McEwen autoradiographic experiments. CI-628 attenuates the sexual differentiation of the rat brain produced by exogenous testosterone (see below).

Toran-Allerand interprets her observations in the light of some general principles by which all neurons appear to develop and form con-

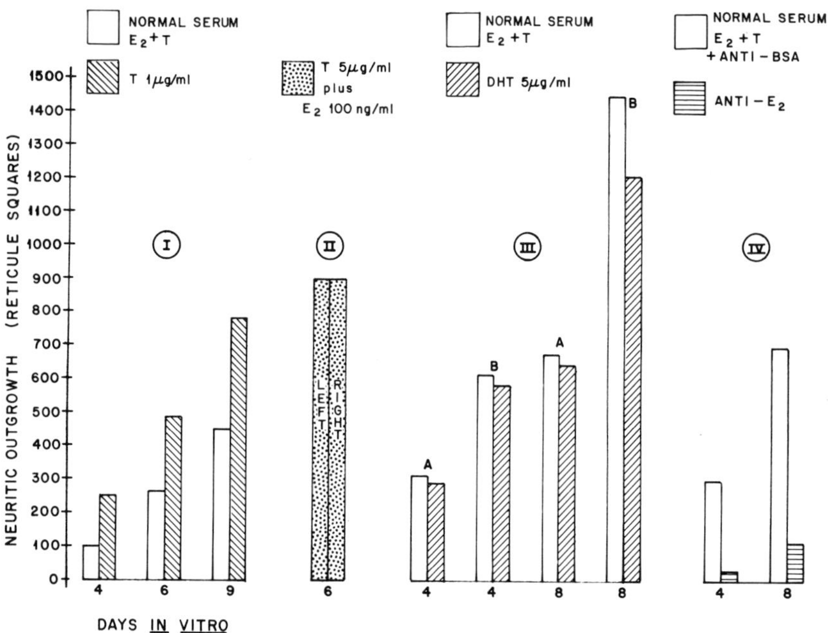

Figure 27. Quantification of the neuritic response in representative homologous pairs of cultures from the preoptic area under various experimental conditions, using a 100-sq. grid of a superimposed ocular reticule. Various examples: I. Induction of neuritic proliferation by exogenous testosterone, 1 μg/ml. II. The effect of exogenous steroid (estradiol plus testosterone) on the neuritic response of right and left halves of a homologous pair of cultures. Note that the growth patterns of both halves are virtually identical and superimposable (901 vs 904 squares). III. The general lack of effect of DHT in inducing a neuritic response in two sets of homologous explant pairs (A and B). Note that the neuritic response of A and B varies considerably in absolute extent, even though the response between the members of each pair is not significantly different. IV. Inhibition of the growth response induced by antibodies to estradiol. [Toran-Allerand]

nections. Differentiation and development of the CNS are based on well-ordered sequences of interlocking phenomena where timing is critical and each aspect is seemingly dependent on the entire sequence of events that have preceded it. Alterations in the timing of sequential phenomena can thus have profound physiological effects without significantly altering the basic morphology, which can thus appear "normal." Morphological differences may exist, however, but be expressed in more subtle ways, such as in the patterns of dendritic differentiation and synaptic organization, which need not be abnormal in themselves but yet result in profound functional differences.

Studies on the ontogeny of dendritic differentiation throughout the CNS (Morest, 1969; Kornguth and Scott, 1972) have led to the concept that patterns of dendritic differentiation and synaptic organization are induced by their afferent axonal input in addition to the cell's genome. Morest (1969) has shown that dendritic differentiation generally follows that of the axon and a close temporal relationship exists between dendritic differentiation and the appearance of afferent endings in their immediate vicinity. Moreover, in studies on the development of the dentate gyrus, Gottlieb and Cowan (1972) have suggested that, since the amount of postsynaptic space available appears to be strictly limited and relatively constant for each neuronal type, the repartition of synaptic sites between different groups of converging axons is determined competitively on a temporal basis. The spatial distribution of synapses, therefore, appears to reflect the differential growth rates of specified axons and the relative number of each axonal category present during synaptogenesis. Patterns of dendritic and synaptic organization have been shown to exhibit considerable postnatal plasticity, however, since environmental factors, such as visual deprivation (Globus and Scheibel, 1967; Parnavelas et al., 1973), and endocrine factors, such as hypothyroidism (Rebière and Legrand, 1972), can modify them.

The timing or rate of axonal development (shown to be critical for the establishment of neuronal interactions in situ) appears to be influenced in vitro by the gonadal steroids. The very neuritic nature of this in vitro response, especially the temporal aspects, suggests that steroid-induced differences in axonal growth patterns may play a role in the neurogenesis of sexual differentiation by so influencing dendritic differentiation and synaptic distribution of target neurons as to result in fundamentally different, gender-specific patterns of neural organization.

The nature of the observed examples of androgen-dependent, sexually dimorphic structures has led to the concept that differences in neuronal circuitry may form the substrate for sexual differentiation. The in vitro observations suggest a possible mechanism by which hormonal effects during morphogenesis could result in the observed differences in the adult brain. All the examples of sexual dimorphism may affect neurons, dendrites, and synapses; these not only constitute the basic components of neuronal networks but may also be viewed as the end result of some aspect of neuritic growth (dendritic branching patterns, synaptic organization, and terminals) and of neuronal development (neuronal nuclear size, neuronal organelles). Thus, steroid-induced changes in neuronal metabolism during the critical period might express themselves morphogenetically in differences in the development of the individual components of neural circuits, the end result of which could produce the observed instances of sexual dimorphism.

Finally, the in vitro observations also suggest that no pattern of sexual differentiation need necessarily be intrinsic to nervous tissue but that male and female patterns may *both* require active induction by steroid. While it is likely that much of the high circulating perinatal levels of estrogen at birth in the rodent are sequestered and functionally inactivated by α-fetoprotein, the degree to which functional activity is reduced is unknown. Rather than representing the passive emergence of the anhormonal state, exposure of the brain to perhaps very low extracellular levels of E_2 in the genetic female during the critical period might induce a given pattern of neural organization. Intraneuronal aromatization of testosterone to E_2, on the other hand, could, perhaps, produce a more localized and concentrated estrogenic effect, and the resultant stimulus to neuritic development might thus induce a different, or male, pattern of neural differentiation. There is also the possibility that, in view of its importance to the differentiation of both sexes, E_2 may have a more general role in neuronal differentiation throughout the CNS; this is possible because of the presence of E_2 receptors in other regions of the CNS during other developmental periods – regions in which aromatization is not present.

Inhibitors of Androgenization in Rodents: Psychotropic Drugs and Antibiotics

Two classes of drugs have been used in an attempt to understand more about the cellular and chemical mechanisms by which sexual differentiation of the rodent brain takes place. One group of drugs includes those that affect neural activity and neurotransmitter metabolism; the other category includes drugs that interfere with DNA, RNA, and protein synthesis.

With respect to psychotropic drugs, Dörner's group (Dörner, 1976, 1977; Dörner et al., 1976, 1977a,c) treated newborn male and female rats with pargyline (a monoamine oxidase inhibitor), reserpine (a depletor of monoamines), and pyridostigmine (an inhibitor of acetylcholinesterase) during the first 2 weeks of life. Treated males, as adults, showed decreased male sexual behavior as a result of pargyline and reserpine treatment and increased male sexual behavior as a result of pyridostigmine treatment. This may have been the result of reduced or enhanced neonatal secretion of testosterone, or it may indicate an independent action of the drugs on neural growth and development. Some hypoplasia of sex organs was observed only in reserpinized, but not in pargylinized, newborn males. Furthermore, male sexual behavior was found to be permanently increased in neonatally pyridostigminized males that showed even a slight hypoplasia of seminal vesicles in neonatal life. These findings suggest that changes of neurotransmitter concentrations and/or turnover rates apparently induced by psychotropic drugs can effect sex-specific brain differentiation by direct action without mediation of sex hormones. Hence, neurotransmitters may be regarded as direct organizers of the brain.* Some indication of the latter possibility came also from the neonatally treated females: pargyline treatment decreased and pyridostigmine treatment increased mounting behavior of females. This effect persisted in the females after ovariectomy and androgen replacement therapy. In addition, the neonatally pyridostigmine-treated females, under androgen replacement therapy, showed enhanced defensive behavior toward males. Under estrogen replacement therapy the pyridostigimine-treated females showed less lordosis behavior toward males, an effect normally seen in neonatally androgenized females. Thus, pyridostigmine may mimic some effects of neonatal androgenization.

Dörner's group has also investigated structural alterations in the brain associated with these various neonatal drug treatments (Dörner et al., 1977c). In adult life, reserpine and pargyline treatment results in increased cell nuclear volumes of nerve cells in the medial and central amygdala. Cell nuclear volumes of treated males, especially those of pargyline-treated males, resemble those of control females. In order to equalize hormonal status of treated males and control females, all animals received testosterone propionate before analysis. Dörner's morphological observations also indicate changes in the number of

*G. Dörner and G. Hinz, manuscript in preparation.

synapses in the striatum radiatum of the hippocampus in neonatally reserpinized adult males compared to controls. Furthermore, significantly increased concentrations of norepinephrine but not of dopamine in the hypothalamus occur in neonatally pargylinized adult males. Significantly reduced levels of norepinephrine were found in the hypothalamus of neonatally pyridostigminized adult males.

Another approach to the question of drug-hormone interaction in the neonate involves attempts to identify agents that can interfere with the action of exogenous androgen in rendering females anovulatory. According to Gorski (1973), however, there are basically three responses of a female rat to a neonatal injection of TP as measured by the incidence of anovulatory sterility: (1) androgenization (large TP doses) – never cycles; (2) delayed anovulatory syndrome (DAS) (low doses of TP) – goes through a few cycles then stops; (3) no effect (extremely low doses of TP) – cycles normally until old age. These three possibilities of neonatal treatment emphasize that one must note the age of the experimental animal at observation. A seemingly ineffective androgenization, as judged by normal ovarian function just after puberty, may well have been effective, as the DAS would demonstrate.

Gorski began by searching for drugs that would obliterate the effects of early androgen exposure. Psychoactive agents such as reserpine, chlorpromazine, and an ovarian and placental steroid, progesterone, were capable of partially blocking an androgenizing dose of TP (30 μg). However, the DAS always ensued, indicating that the action of TP had only been attenuated (Arai and Gorski, 1968c). Interestingly, an agent that has purported blocking effects on androgenization when given after the critical period is over is chlorpromazine. According to Ladosky and co-workers (1970), giving chlorpromazine to 10-day-old males rendered them able to support ovulation as adults. It seems unlikely that progesterone could be the natural antiandrogen.

The failure of a relatively high dose of progesterone (2500 μg), given concurrently with TP to inhibit androgenization, suggests that this hormone is not a natural antiandrogen that might be expected to protect the female rat against the prenatal hormonal environment. In fact, since this same dose of progesterone can apparently induce the anovulatory condition itself, it may be that the attenuation of androgenization that has been observed is the consequence of a nonspecific, perhaps anesthetic, effect of progesterone (Arai and Gorski, 1968c).

Finally, it should be noted that the postnatal differentiation of the rat brain may represent a species-specific exception to the more common pattern of differentiation in utero, thus, in an environment presumably rich in progesterone.

Since barbiturates had been employed to block ovulation in adults, they were tried in neonates, and both pentobarbital and phenobarbital administered acutely with TP were able to provide long-lasting protection from androgenization, with little occurrence of the DAS (Arai and Gorski, 1968a,c; Gorski, 1974a). However, this effect might have nothing to do with the anesthetic properties of the drugs, but rather could reflect a direct competition with T for the cerebral aromatase system, a system known to contain cytochrome P450. The role of aromatization will be considered again below. The protective effect of pentobarbital could be counteracted with Metrazol, a convulsant drug, but Metrazol itself had no effect on androgenization.

The use of drugs in another approach is to study possible genomic involvement in sexual differentiation by means of inhibitors of DNA, RNA, and protein synthesis. Again using anovulatory sterility as the end point of androgen action, Kobayashi and Gorski (1970) found that subcutaneous administration of actinomycin D or puromycin 2 to 4 hours after administration of 20 μg of TP to 5-day-old female rats reduced significantly the number of anovulatory animals on day 45. All TP-treated animals were anovulatory at day 90, however, indicating that the antibiotics were only partially effective. In a subsequent study, Gorski and Shryne (1972) reported that intrahypothalamic cycloheximide (in cocoa butter) on day 5 attenuated the effects of 30 μg of TP on anovulatory sterility measured on day 45, but again had no effect on sterility on day 90. Other antibiotics, given intracranially, were ineffective. Barnea and Lindner (1972) found that intrahypothalamic treatment with protein synthesis inhibitors, hydroxyurea and 5-bromodeoxyuridine, were ineffective in blocking TP-induced anovulatory sterility. In contrast to Gorski and Shryne (1972), Barnea and Lindner (1972) used a higher dose of TP (100 μg) and infused the inhibitors in a large volume of saline (10 μl).

A report by Salaman (1974) indicates a successful attenuation of TP-induced anovulatory sterility measured at days 80 to 90 by RNA, protein, and DNA synthesis inhibitors given subcutaneously on postnatal day 4 together with TP and again 6 hours later. Hydroxyurea, a DNA synthesis inhibitor with additional effects on overall RNA synthesis, and α-amanitin, an inhibitor of "messenger" RNA synthesis, attenuated effects of 30, 80, and 200 μg of TP. Puromycin and actinomycin D were generally less effective in the doses used. It should also be noted that α-amanitin and hydroxyurea were, by themselves, ineffective in inducing anovulatory sterility.

In an attempt to implicate further DNA synthesis and cell division, Salaman (1977) administered colchicine, a mitotic inhibitor, to 4-day-old female Wistar rats and observed some protection from the defeminizing effects of 80 μg of TP on neuroendocrine function. Colchicine was more effective when given with and after TP than when given before it. As promising as these experiments are, the following questions arise: (1) Are the primary effects ascribed to these inhibitors actually the reasons for their effects, or are other metabolic actions responsible? (2) Is the brain necessarily the site of action of these drugs in view of the lesser success of intracranial application of the drugs? (3) What is the critical exposure time to TP during which such drugs must be effective?

With respect to the first question, it is at least possible to point to alterations in RNA and protein metabolism in the brain associated with gonadal secretion or gonadal steroid administration during the first days of postnatal life. In one study, testosterone administration to 2-day-old female rats significantly *decreased* within 4 hours the incorporation of ^{3}H-uridine into RNA in all brain regions *except* the anterior hypothalamus and medial amygdala (Clayton et al., 1970). The investigators attributed special significance to the sparing action in the anterior hypothalamus and amygdala in view of the presumed importance of these areas in the regulation of gonadotropin secretion. Westley and Salaman (1975) also observed 25 to 50% decreases in ^{3}H-uridine incorporation into hypothalamic RNA lasting from 2 to 10 hours after the administration of 1 mg of testosterone propionate to 4-day-old female rats.

Another study reported increases in ^{3}H-leucine incorporation into neurons of the arcuate nucleus 24 hours after castration of full-term fetal male rats (Nakai et al., 1971). These investigators preferred to interpret their results as indicating that "the hypothalamic-pituitary-testicular axis begins to function before birth." Another brief report indicated increased incorporation of ^{35}S-methionine in the thalamus and amygdala 12 and 24 hours after TP treatment of 3-day-old female rats (Darrah et al., 1961). In none of the above-mentioned cases is there any compelling evidence that these changes reflect early events in sexual differentiation; but the evidence does indicate that the neonatal brain responds, directly or indirectly, to androgen treatment by altered RNA and protein metabolism.

Brain Sites of Androgen Action

Direct evidence for androgen effects on brain differentiation (see question 2 in preceding section) comes from implantation of testosterone into the brains of neonatal female rats. Nadler (1968, 1972, 1973) found that TP implants in the region of the ventromedial and arcuate nuclei of 5-day-old female rats were most effective in inducing anovulatory sterility and reducing female sexual receptivity. Subcutaneous implants of TP were ineffective as were TP implants in a great many other brain regions. Hayashi and Gorski (1974) reported anovulatory sterility from implantation of TP bilaterally into both ventromedial-arcuate and anterior hypothalamic sites of 3-day-old female rats. Using a removable implant, they found that 48 to 72 hours of exposure to TP were most effective, and this result implies that drugs that are used to attenuate TP effects must be applied so as to act for a considerable length of time. Thus, with respect to question 3 above, inhibitor experiments performed thus far may not have produced a long enough duration of macromolecular synthesis inhibition to be completely successful.

Gorski's findings of a 2- to 3-day minimal exposure time for complete androgenization with intracranial implants of T contrast with his earlier demonstration that barbiturates (Arai and Gorski, 1968a) and an antiandrogen, cyproterone acetate (Arai and Gorski, 1968b), given systemically, only block action of systemic TP when given within 6 to 12 hours of the steroid. The discrepancy is not easy to explain. It may be, however, that the faster action of systemic TP is related to its rapid access to all areas of the brain and the slower action of intracranial T is an indication of diffusion from the implantation site to other brain regions. This explanation implies that there are multiple sites of androgen action in the developing rat brain and suggests that the search for sexually dimorphic brain regions (see above discussion) should be widened to other parts of the brain. Recently, Christensen and Gorski (1978) have reported temporally, hormonally, and spatially specific consequences of the neonatal implantation of E_2 or T within the hypothalamic-preoptic area. Although in this study steroid implants within the mesencephalic reticular formation were without effect, other observations have prompted Gorski (1974b) to speculate that this region of the brain may also be altered by androgen neonatally. Definitive studies of androgen action require the identification of primary and secondary sites of action specific to known functional, biochemical, or morphological alterations.

Alterations in the Length of the Critical Period

The existence of a hormonal critical period during the time in brain development of extensive synapse formation and neurogenesis indicates that cell proliferation and growth may be influenced by gonadal steroids. As far as cell proliferation is concerned, the efficacy of colchicine (a mitotic blocking agent but also an inhibitor of axonal transport) in attenuating the defeminizing effects of TP treatment in female rats may be interpreted as indicating a stimulation by TP of cell proliferation (Salaman, 1977). On the other hand, most, if not all, of the cell proliferation within the hypothalamus and preoptic area of the rat brain has ceased by 16 or 17 days of gestation, before the critical period has commenced (Ifft, 1972). With regard to neuronal growth and maturation, there are studies with thyroid hormone that indicate that the critical period for gonadal steroid action is related to the state of neural maturation. Hypothyroidism in the early postnatal period retards myelinization and development of the neuropil and reduces synapse formation, although it does not decrease cell number; hyperthyroidism at birth decreases total cell number, facilitates myelinization, and transiently increases synapse formation (see Grave, 1977). With respect to sexual differentiation, hypothyroidism at birth prolongs the critical period of susceptibility of female rats to the defeminizing effects of TP (Kikuyama, 1969). Hyperthyroidism shortly after birth, on the other hand, shortens the critical period of susceptibility of TP (Kikuyama, 1966; Phelps and Sawyer, 1976).

Gorski described experiments on septally lesioned adult rats that suggest that steroids influence neural plasticity long after the neonatal critical period is over. Septal lesions render females, but not males, more sensitive to estrogen priming as measured by lordosis behavior. However, if male rats are exposed to EB for 10 days immediately after the septal lesion, they also exhibit a prolonged (presumably permanent) and marked increase in behavioral sensitivity to estrogen (Nance et al., 1975, 1977). Hypothyroidism in septally lesioned males also increases their sensitivity to EB priming in the display of lordosis (Nance et al., 1977). Gorski interprets these results as indicating an involvement of both gonadal steroids and thyroid hormone in some dynamic process associated with recovery from brain lesions, a process that may have certain similarities with sexual differentiation.

Another aspect of steroid-related plasticity in adult rats was described by Gorski. As indicated above, if a female rat is treated on day 5 of life with low doses of TP (10 μg), the DAS ensues at around day 70. It can be demonstrated that these animals undergo normal and inducible LH surges before DAS ensues, while, after DAS onset, normal LH surges cease, nor can they be induced. If, however, a potential DAS animal is ovariectomized prior to DAS onset, the ability to demonstrate an induced LH surge will not disappear. This effect of ovariectomy can be reversed with EB or TP replacement (Harlan and Gorski, 1978). These results, in conjunction with the fact that the normal female eventually ceases to cycle at a later age, supports the notion that early exposure to androgen is actually accelerating the aging process (Swanson and van der Werff ten Bosch, 1964). Dörner actually has data supporting this notion, demonstrating that life-spans of normal males and androgenized females are shorter than those of neonatally castrated males and normal females. This also relates to Gerall's work, which demonstrates that a potential DAS rat will continue to ovulate for increasingly longer periods of time if she is allowed to mate, become pregnant, give birth, and lactate. Studies are in progress to determine whether the delay in the onset of androgen-induced sterility is due to increased levels of progesterone or prolactin. Gorski's observation that prolactin changes markedly during DAS onset encourages further research on the role of this hormone in maintaining normal cyclic ovarian capacity. Gerall's conclusion is that prolactin is important for the maintenance of normal endocrine function, which is supported by Gorski's observation that prolactin changes quite markedly during DAS onset (Harlan and Gorski, 1977).

Metabolism of Steroid Hormones by Brain Tissue

The importance of intracellular metabolites of gonadal steroid hormones in mediating the action of the parent hormone was first recognized in relation to dihydrotestosterone: This metabolite was shown to be produced from testosterone by 5α-reduction in target organs such as the prostate, to bind to the androgen receptor protein, to concentrate in the cell nuclei, and to have in some bioassays potency equal to or greater than that of testosterone (Wilson and Gloyna, 1970). That dihydrotestosterone formation not only occurs but is essential for mediating some of the androgenic actions of testosterone is illustrated by the incomplete masculinization seen in individuals with an inherited defect characterized by a greatly diminished capacity for 5α-reduction of testosterone (Imperato-McGinley and Peterson, 1976). Formation of active metabolites in target cells from circulating prehormones has since been established as an important general principle in steroid hormone action. It applies to various target organs, including the CNS, to a number of metabolites of testosterone besides dihydrotestosterone, and to prehormones other than testosterone.

The function of active metabolite formation within target tissues may be viewed as a means to diversify the action of a single steroid hormone by producing, in situ, agents able to interact at different points in intracellular metabolism. It may provide a mechanism for achieving high concentrations of specific metabolites at discrete sites and for modulating hormone action through the regulation of the activity of the metabolizing enzymes. Not surprisingly, the CNS may prove to be the target organ in which these possibilities are most extensively exploited.

Figure 28 shows the major metabolic pathways by which the various potentially active metabolites of testosterone are formed. Brain tissue has been shown to have the ability to carry out all of these metabolic steps (Denef et al., 1973; Fishman and Norton, 1975; Naftolin et al., 1975b; Martini, 1976; Kao et al., 1977; Weisz et al., 1978). Testosterone can be channeled basically into two directions, one involving 5α-reduction and the other aromatization. In the CNS, enzyme reactions for both metabolic reactions have been found to be concentrated primarily in the hypothalamus and amygdala, providing presumptive evidence for their role in neuroendocrine regulation.

The first product of 5α-reduction of testosterone is dihydrotestosterone, the prototype of the metabolite that can mediate the action of its precursor or parent hormone. Dihydrotestosterone can be further reduced at the 3α or 3β position. There are some indications from recent studies that the 3β-reduced metabolite, 5α-androstan-3β-17β-diol (3β-androstandiol), may have actions distinct from those of

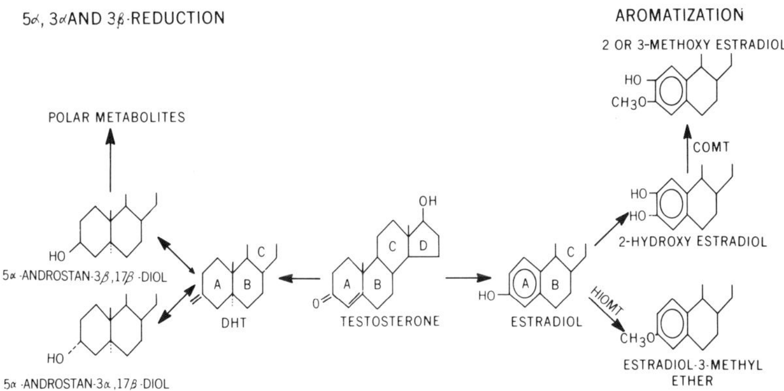

Figure 28. Major metabolic pathways by which various potentially active metabolites of testosterone are formed. [Weisz]

dihydrotestosterone (Robel et al., 1971; Kao and Weisz, 1975; Rennie et al., 1977). Since this metabolite, unlike dihydrotestosterone, does not bind to the androgen receptor protein or concentrate in the cell nuclei, any action it may have must be initiated through an extranuclear mechanism.

Establishing if 5α-androstan-3α, 17βdiol is biologically active in its own right presents problems, since 3α-reduction appears to be readily reversible in most tissues, including the CNS (Kao et al., 1977). Consequently, 3α-androstandiol reaching these tissues should, theoretically, be readily reconvertible to dihydrotestosterone. In contrast, formation of dihydrotestosterone from 3β-androstandiol in the CNS and the anterior pituitary is likely to be restricted because of the rapid conversion of 3β-androstandiol to polar metabolites (Kao et al., 1977).

The second major route of testosterone metabolism involves aromatization of the A-ring of the steroid. This results in the formation of estradiol, a highly potent steroid. Androstenedione, which can be formed in the CNS from testosterone, can be converted by the same aromatizing enzyme system to estrone (Weisz and Gibbs, 1974a,b; Naftolin et al., 1975b). The estrogens can be further metabolized by hydroxylation at carbon 2. This metabolic step confers a catechol structure on the aromatic A-ring of the steroid molecule and thereby opens up a number of new possibilities for biochemical interaction. Through their catechol structure, the 2-hydroxylated or catechol estrogens can serve as substrates for catechol-*O*-methyltransferase and act as competitive inhibitors of the inactivation of catecholamines by this enzyme (Breuer and Köster, 1975; Lloyd et al., 1978). More recently, catechol estrogens have been shown to inhibit, in vitro, the activity of tyrosine hydroxylase, the enzyme that catalyzes the presumed rate-limiting step in catecholamine biosynthesis (Lloyd and Weisz, 1978). Thus, through this metabolite, estrogens and therefore their C-19 precursors, testosterone or androstenedione, may interact directly with enzymes regulating the biosynthesis and inactivation of dopamine and norepinephrine to influence the turnover of these catecholamines. The significance of these intriguing possibilities for neuroendocrine regulation in vivo will now have to be examined critically. Whether the catechol structure of the 2-hydroxylated estrogens permits them to interact with receptors for catecholamines has not yet been tested. All of these actions of the catechol estrogens would operate without involving the nucleus and therefore without influencing, at least directly, genomic function.

Hydroxylation of estrogens at carbon 2, however, does not abolish their original steroid characteristics. Catechol estrogens can still bind to the estrogen receptor protein with an affinity only about one order of magnitude less than that of their respective estrogen precursors and be translocated to the nucleus (Davies et al., 1975; Martucci and Fishman 1976). On this basis it has been proposed that catechol estrogens may act as antiestrogens by competing for the receptor. The duration of receptor occupancy by catechol estrogens and the influence they have on receptor turnover will, however, have to be determined before it is possible to decide if the 2-hydroxylated estrogens qualify as antiestrogens (Anderson et al., 1975; Clark et al., 1977; Katzenellenbogen et al., 1977).

The ability of catechol estrogens to influence gonadotropin regulation has now been demonstrated in a few studies (Naftolin et al., 1975a; Parvizi and Ellendorf, 1975; Gethmann and Knuppen, 1976). Whether the findings reflect physiological or pharmacological actions of the catechol estrogens is as yet unknown. Nor have the mechanisms through which these effects are achieved been examined. Finally, estradiol itself can undergo *O*-methylation by hydroxyindole-*O*-methyltransferase in a manner analogous to the *O*-methylation of the catechol estrogens by catechol-*O*-methyltransferase (Weisz et al., 1978). Whether this confers on estrogens the potential to interact with the indole pathway remains to be determined.

In the mammalian CNS the hypothalamus and the amygdala appear to be the sites of maximum concentration of the enzymes that catalyze 5α-reduction and aromatization of testosterone, as well as 2-hydroxylation of estrogens (Weisz and Gibbs, 1974a; Naftolin et al., 1975b; Fishman and Norton, 1975; Martini, 1976). The testosterone-metabolizing potential of the CNS is probably established early in development. In fact, this potential, as determined by in vitro studies and on a per mg basis, is higher in fetal and neonatal life than in the adult (Weisz and Gibbs, 1974a; Naftolin et al., 1975b; George et al., 1978).

More detailed mapping of the exact sites in the hypothalamus and amygdala where these metabolizing enzymes are concentrated has begun only recently. This information may provide clues to the functions with which these metabolites are associated and is needed for designing more critical experiments on the factors that regulate the activity of the enzymes. A sufficiently sensitive assay has been developed for the aromatizing enzyme system to make it possible to measure the level of its activity in punch biopsy specimens from individual rats. The findings of Kobayashi and Reed (1977), who used this approach, are shown in Table 5. Several interesting points are illustrated by their study. The enzyme activity clearly is not distributed uniformly but is severalfold higher in some brain nuclei than in others. Significant concentrations of estradiol may build up in relation to certain neuronal populations even though the overall conversion of testosterone to estradiol in homogenates of whole hypothalami of adult rats is less than 1%. In general, the level of aromatase activity is higher in males than in females. This sex difference is most obvious when nuclei with the highest activity in males are compared with those in females. Castration reduces the aromatase activity of males to the level of females. The only exception is the medial cortical amygdaloid nucleus. Enzyme activity in this site is comparably high in the two sexes and is unaffected by orchidectomy. Clearly, these sex differences and the response to castration would be much less evident if larger tissue specimens were used. Selmanoff and co-workers (1977) studied both aromatase and 5α-reductase activity in pooled punch biopsy specimens from hypothalamic and amygdaloid nuclei of adult rats. Though there are some differences in the details of the findings from the studies, perhaps because Selmanoff and co-workers used gonadectomized and adrenalectomized rats, the same general principles are evident. An important additional finding in their study is disassociation between the aromatase and the 5α-reductase activity. The results from these two

TABLE 5

Regional Distribution of Steroid Aromatase Activity in Male and Female Rats [Kobayashi and Reed, 1977]

Region	Male	Female	Castrated male
Preoptic			
N. preopticus medialis	301 ± 67 (6)	99 ± 18 (6)*	127 ± 16 (6)*
N. preopticus lateralis	23 ± 7 (6)	9 ± 2 (5)	
N. preopticus periventricularis	265 ± 37 (6)	143 ± 12 (6)**	
N. preopticus suprachiasmatis	39 ± 8 (5)	10 ± 2 (5)**	12 ± 4 (4)*
Organum vasculosum lamina	70 ± 20 (2)	41 ± 6 (2)	56 ± 7 (2)
Hypothalamus			
N. hypothalamicus anterior	105 ± 26 (6)	30 ± 7 (6)*	
N. supraopticus	13 ± 1 (3)	10 ± 2 (3)	
N. paraventricularis	21 ± 2 (4)	20 ± 5 (4)	
Median eminence	16 ± 2 (4)	9 ± 5 (4)	
N. arcuatus	26 ± 2 (6)	20 ± 5 (6)	
N. ventromedialis	63 ± 7 (6)	55 ± 3 (6)	34 ± 6 (6)**
Limbic			
N. septi	52 ± 17 (6)	18 ± 5 (6)	
N. accumbens	41 ± 15 (6)	28 ± 2 (6)	24 ± 3 (6)
N. amygdaloideus medialis	290 ± 90 (6)	269 ± 39 (6)	298 ± 64 (6)
N. amygdaloideus centralis	146 ± 90 (6)	50 ± 5 (6)	
N. amygdaloideus corticalis	26 ± 4 (6)	13 ± 2 (4)*	12 ± 2 (6)**

Figures are in pmole of estrone /h/g of protein; mean ± S.E.M.
Significant differences compared to intact males determined by t test (* $P < .05$, ** $P < .01$).

pioneering studies are generally consistent with results of in vivo studies in which the conversion of ^{3}H-testosterone to ^{3}H-estradiol and ^{3}H-dihydrotestosterone was monitored at the tissue and cell nuclear level (Lieberburg and McEwen, 1977). The main finding of this latter study is that ^{3}H-estradiol predominates as a metabolite of ^{3}H-testosterone in the amygdala (see Table 5 for comparison) and ^{3}H-dihydrotestosterone predominates as a metabolite in the pituitary. Further investigation of the anatomical distribution of the aromatizing enzymes in the brain must be conducted to determine whether all estrogen-sensitive neurons have associated aromatase activity or whether only a select subgroup has this property.

The evidence discussed so far points to there being at least four biologically active metabolites of testosterone, i.e., dihydrotestosterone, 3β-androstandiol, estradiol, and 2-hydroxyestradiol, that may be formed in discrete sites in the CNS in significant concentrations to participate in mediating the androgenic action of the parent hormone on this target organ. In addition, at least one of the metabolites, 2-hydroxyestradiol, may act through two quite distinct mechanisms, because it resembles the catecholamines as well as the classical steroidal estrogens. What role does each of these metabolites actually have in mediating the diverse effects of androgens on brain differentiation and function?

There are obvious difficulties in designing definitive experiments to answer this question. Data on the effects of the metabolites administered systemically could be misleading. By using this approach, the levels of the administered hormone reaching the relevant sites cannot be controlled nor can its action be restricted and be as selective as that which may be achieved by the discretely localized enzyme systems. Useful experimental tools are, however, becoming available in the form of agents that can specifically block the formation of one or the other metabolite or block the uptake of the metabolite by steroid receptor protein. Agents that block aromatization of testosterone have now been used to demonstrate the importance of aromatization for defeminization of sexual behavior by endogenous testosterone in the newborn male rat (Vreebrug et al., 1977) and masculinization and defeminization of this behavior in the newborn female rat by exogenous testosterone (McEwen et al., 1977).* This will be discussed further below.

Role of Dihydrotestosterone and Estradiol as Mediators of Testosterone Action

Assessments of the relative importance of aromatization and 5α-reduction in the action of T on brain function have involved several interrelated strategies. One strategy, as summarized by Gerall, is to give androgens that are not aromatizable, in an attempt to mimic effects of T replacement therapy. Dihydrotestosterone is the most frequently used because of its potency in stimulating the growth of the male reproductive tract. There are some species in which DHT can maintain or prolong male sexual behavior after castration: the rhesus monkey, the guinea pig, the hamster, and the rabbit. There are other species in

*J. Weisz and I.L. Ward, unpublished data.

which DHT has little, if any, effect; but aromatizable androgens, like T or androstenedione, are effective, e.g., the Japanese quail and the rat. The largest number of studies has been done on the rat, and, while most investigators have not observed effects of DHT, a few have found some indication that DHT prolongs the period of sexual activity after castration. Luttge and Hall (1973a,b) have found that DHT can maintain male behavior in one strain of mice, Swiss-Webster, but not in another, Cb-1. Such observations with DHT have led to another strategy, namely, to give both estradiol and DHT at doses that are not effective when given separately. This is based on the notion that DHT may be needed to maintain reproductive tract function and E_2 to activate central mechanisms. A number of reports for the rat indicate that EB plus DHTP maintains male sexual behavior (Baum and Vreeburg, 1973; Larsson et al., 1973; Feder et al., 1974; Luttge et al., 1975). Another report indicates that DHT may act centrally as well as peripherally in the rat, because DHT-E_2 synergism is observed even in rats in which the genitalia have been locally anesthetized (Baum et al., 1974). There is another finding that the synergism does not work in adrenalectomized (ADX) rats, which would indicate that estrogen stimulation of the adrenal may be involved. On the other hand, Luttge does find synergism of E_2 plus DHT in castrated ADX mice (Luttge et al., 1975). Davis and Barfield (1979) have observed that highly localized implants of EB in the POA, together with peripheral administration of DHT, are very effective in restoring male sexual behavior in castrated rats.

There are certain parallels between the story of aromatization and the activation of male sexual behavior and the story of aromatization and brain sexual differentiation. In species where DHT activates male sexual behavior, such as guinea pig and rhesus monkey, DHT also appears capable of organizing it (Alsum and Goy, 1974; Phoenix, 1974; Goldfoot and van der Werff ten Bosch, 1975).* In species where the activational effect of DHT is less pronounced or negligible, e.g., rat, mouse, and hamster, DHT is generally without effect in organizing it, but aromatizable androgens and estrogens are effective. In the rat, DHT administration in neonatal life suppresses gonadotropin (and therefore T) secretion and is capable of blocking the normal sexual differentiation in the male by this process (Korenbrot et al., 1975). At the same time, DHT treatment results in a normally responsive male reproductive tract, and, given to females, does not appear to have a permanent effect

*Also C.H. Phoenix and R.W. Goy, unpublished observations.

on the ovary. DHT is not, in the rat, able to promote either masculinization of male sexual behavior or defeminization (i.e., suppression of female behavior) or ovulation, in contrast to T and E_2, which are both effective in these regards. Gerall and collaborators (1975) noted that several instances of inhibition of lordosis later in life by neonatal DHT treatment may be explained by its effect on the vagina. They found that the DHT effects disappeared when they covered the vagina of the treated and control females with tape and tested them with males.

It is important to understand the underlying reasons for the species differences in the effectiveness of DHT. Since DHT metabolism is rapid in the rat and slower in rhesus monkey, it is conceivable that some of the ineffectiveness of DHT in the former and effectiveness in the latter species may be explained by the amount of DHT that actually reaches target cells in the brain. On the other hand, it is likely that some of the differences are actually those in target tissue sensitivity, i.e., the cells that respond to hormone and undergo developmental changes that underlie sexual differentiation contain different kinds of receptors in estrogen-responsive and DHT-responsive species.

The effects of neonatal estrogen treatment of rats – generally speaking to defeminize female behavior and, perhaps, also to enhance male behavioral patterns – are, nevertheless, complicated by other effects. Zadina and collaborators (1979) have found that neonatal treatment of male rats with EB delays the age of testicular descent. So, also, do high doses of TP, perhaps by being converted to estradiol. Neonatal EB treatment also reduces the response of prostate and seminal vesicles in adult castrates exposed to TP. Perhaps as a result of these effects, neonatal EB treatment does, in males, reduce somewhat the degree to which masculine sexual behavior can be elicited in adulthood. In neonatal life concurrent administration of EB with DHT ameliorates the effects of EB alone and results in larger percentages of treated males showing ejaculation as adults. Gerall speculates that it is an effect of EB on penis development, which is counteracted by DHT, that accounts for these results.

Role of Aromatization in Rat Brain Sexual Differentiation

Several kinds of evidence point to the involvement of aromatization in the sexual differentiation of the rat brain. First, there is the aforementioned conversion of ^{3}H-testosterone (or androstanedione) to ^{3}H-estradiol (or estrone) and the retention of ^{3}H-estradiol by cell nuclei in the hypothalamus and limbic areas of the neonatal rat brain (Reddy et al., 1974; Weisz and Gibbs, 1974a; Lieberburg and McEwen, 1975; Lieberburg et al., 1977b). Hypothalamic estrogen receptors of 4-day-old male rats are partially occupied by androgen-derived estradiol (Westley and Salaman, 1976, 1977; Lieberburg et al., 1979). The cerebral cortex does not contain aromatizing enzymes and cortical estrogen receptors are not occupied by endogenous steroids in 4-day-old male rats (Westley and Salaman, 1976, 1977; Lieberburg et al., 1979). In this connection it is noteworthy that intrahypothalamic implants of estradiol (Döcke and Dörner, 1975; Marcus et al., 1977; Christensen and Gorski, 1978), as well as of T (Wagner et al., 1966; Nadler, 1973; Hayashi and Gorski, 1974), into newborn female rats leads to anovulatory sterility in adult life.

Second, there is the demonstration of cell nuclear and soluble estrogen receptors in brains of newborn rats. These receptors (see next section) have a specificity that parallels the action spectrum of steroids, insofar as it is presently known, in inducing brain sexual differentiation. Proof that aromatization actually plays a significant role in brain sexual differentiation requires that one prevent the effect of exogenous T in females and endogenous T in males by agents that either block aromatization or prevent access of estrogen to intracellular receptor sites.

With respect to inhibitors of aromatization, Clemens (1974) has reported some success in blocking the masculinizing effects of T given to castrated, newborn hamsters by means of pentobarbital and SKF-525A, which may decrease aromatization by competing for microsomal hydroxylating enzymes. More definitive results have recently been obtained by Lieberburg and co-workers (1977b), using a steroid inhibitor of aromatization, androst-1,4,6-triene-3,17-dione (ATD). Implantation of silastic capsules of ATD into 4-day-old female rats reduced by more than 80% cell nuclear levels of $^3HE_2$ derived from an injection of ^3HT (Table 6). Tissue levels of $^3HE_2$ and ^3H-estrone were also reduced, indicating that aromatization is affected. Tissue and cell nuclear levels of ^3HT and ^3HDHT were unaltered by ATD treatment, and ATD did not interfere with the cell nuclear retention of ^3H-diethylstilbestrol, indicating that it is neutral with respect to the estrogen receptor mechanism (Lieberburg et al., 1977b). ATD treatment of newborn male rats feminized them with respect to their ability to display lordosis behavior as adults, and ATD treatment of females also given T blocked the defeminizing effects of T on lordosis behavior and on ovulation (Table 7, Part 1; McEwen et al., 1977). Similar results have

TABLE 6

Effect of CI-628 or ATD Pretreatment on in vivo Formed Testosterone Metabolites Recovered from Neonatal Female Brain Homogenates and Purified Cell Nuclear Fractions [Lieberburg et al., 1977b]

Pre-treatment	Fraction	Total	A_0	Diol	T	DHT	A	a	E_2	E_1
Control	WH	631 ± 64	58.1 ± 15.6	16.6 ± 2.0	69.5 ± 7.6	13.9 ± 2.5	30.2 ± 3.1	4.57 ± 0.72	1.40 ± 0.04	0.83 ± 0.09
	N	6.43 ± 0.57	0.58 ± 0.07	0.29 ± 0.05	1.54 ± 0.16	0.65 ± 0.05	0.64 ± 0.08	0.23 ± 0.02	1.78 ± 0.35	U
CI-628	WH	681 ± 49	64.2 ± 14.7	19.0 ± 1.0	76.6 ± 4.6	14.2 ± 0.8	33.8 ± 2.8	5.04 ± 0.52	1.19 ± 0.12	1.01 ± 0.09
	N	5.37 ± 0.59	0.57 ± 0.05	0.30 ± 0.05	1.52 ± 0.14	0.63 ± 0.04	0.33 ± 0.09*	0.21 ± 0.01	0.36 ± 0.03**, §	U
ATD	WH	646 ± 80	68.4 ± 18.3	14.3 ± 3.0	83.4 ± 12.9	20.0 ± 2.6	37.6 ± 5.5	8.71 ± 1.49*	0.82 ± 0.06 ***, §	0.08 ± 0.04 ***, §§
	N	4.71 ± 0.37*	0.59 ± 0.07	0.30 ± 0.05	1.50 ± 0.18	0.72 ± 0.07	0.36 ± 0.11	0.34 ± 0.06	0.32 ± 0.06 ***, §	U

WH = whole tissue homogenate, N = purified cell nuclei. Radioactivity was analyzed according to the method of Lieberburg and McEwen (1977), which involves double isotope dilution, toluene extraction, phenolic separation, separation of neutral steroids (androgens) on silica gel plates with two developments in $CHCl_3$-ether 20:1 (v/v), methylation of estrogens, and separation of estrogen-3-methyl ethers on silica gel plates with one development in benzene-ethanol 95:5 (v/v). A_0 = radioactivity recovered from the origin of the neutral steroids plate ($CHCl_3$-ether 20:1), probably representing very polar androgens; Diol = radioactivity recovered from the spot containing 3α- + 3β-androstanediol; T = testosterone; DHT = 5α-dihydrotestosterone; A = androstenedione; a = androstanedione; E_2 = estradiol-17β; E_1 = estrone. U signifies undetectable.

* $P < 0.05$, ** $P < 0.01$, *** $P < 0.001$, significantly different from control (t-test).

§ $P < 0.025$, §§ $P < 0.005$, significantly different from control (Dunnett).

TABLE 7

Part 1. Effect of Neonatal Treatment with T and ATD on Sexual Differentiation in Male and Female Rats [McEwen et al., 1977]

Treat-ment	Number of rats	Day of vaginal opening	Body wt (Days 75-76)	Ovarian wt/ body wt (mg/g)	Corpora lutea/ section	LQ[1]
Female						
CH:CH[2]	10	39 ± 1[3]	253 ± 5	1.21 ± .08	5.9 ± .8	89 ± 3
CH:T	17	12/16 (NO)[4]	306 ± 6*	0.53 ± .04*	0.03 ± .03*	18 ± 7*
ATD:CH	18	39 ± 1	261 ± 5	1.32 ± .05	7.8 ± .4	86 ± 4
ATD:T	14	41 ± 2	256 ± 5	1.30 ± .05	6.6 ± .6	82 ± 5
Male						
CH	20	–	334 ± 11	–	–	0(0/20)
ATD	18	–	330 ± 7	–	–	90(16/18**)

[1] Lordosis quotient. Number of rats showing lordosis response is indicated within parentheses.
[2] CH: cholesterol.
[3] Mean ± SEM.
[4] NO: vaginal opening did not occur in 12/17 animals.
* Different from CH:CH by Newman-Keuls test: $P < 0.01$.
** Different from CH by chi-square test: $P < 0.005$.

Part 2. Effect of Neonatal Treatment with CI628 on Sexual Differentiation in Male and Female Rats

Treat-ment	Number of rats	Day of vaginal opening	Body wt (Days 76-80)	Ovarian wt/ body wt (mg/g)	Corpora lutea/ section	LQ
Female						
Control	23	39 ± 1	261 ± 4	1.47 ± .06	6.4 ± .5	81 ± 3
CI628	19	35 ± 1*	276 ± 7	1.32 ± .06	4.0 ± .6**	66 ± 5***
Male						
Control	24	–	347 ± 10	–	–	26 ± 5
CI628	34	–	346 ± 7	–	–	53 ± 5*

Mean ± SEM.
* $P < 0.001$, students t test.
** $P < 0.01$, students t test.
*** $P < 0.02$, students t test.

TABLE 7 *(continued)*

Part 3. Effect of Neonatal Treatment with TP and CI628 on Ovarian Function and Lordosis Quotient

Treat-ment	Number of rats	Day of vaginal opening	Body wt (Day 75)	Ovarian wt/ body wt (mg/g)	Corpora lutea/ section	LQ
Control	19	38 ± 1[1]	205 ± 6	1.85 ± .10	5.5 ± .6	73 ± 4
TP	19	35 ± 1**	206 ± 2	0.90 ± .05*	0.1 ± .1*	35 ± 5***
TP + CI	16	35 ± 1**	211 ± 4	1.01 ± .15*	1.2 ± .7**	52 ± 7**

[1] Mean ± SEM.
* Different from control by Newman-Keuls test: $P < 0.01$.
** Different from control by Newman-Keuls test: $P < 0.05$.
*** TP vs TP + CI by Newman-Keuls: $P < 0.05$.

been reported by Vreeburg and co-workers (1977), using ATD, and by Booth (1977a), using a related steroid, androst-4-ene-3,6,17-trione.

With respect to inhibitors of estrogen receptors, there have been reports of success in preventing defeminization of female rats by neonatal testosterone propionate, by using a nonsteroidal estrogen antagonist, MER-25 (Doughty and McDonald, 1974). MER-25 also antagonizes the defeminizing action of a synthetic estrogen, RU-2858, on brain sexual differentiation (Doughty et al., 1975b). There have also been three reports of failures to obtain such antagonistic effects with MER-25 (Brown-Grant, 1974; Gottlieb et al., 1974; Hayashi, 1974), which may be explained by the poor solubility and limited effectiveness of this estrogen antagonist (Ruh and Ruh, 1974).

Recent experiments by McEwen and co-workers (1977) with a more potent antiestrogen, CI-628, support the successful MER-25 experiments. CI-628 treatment of neonatal male rats feminized them with respect to the display of lordosis as adults (Table 7, Part 2). CI-628 treatment of newborn females also treated with TP attenuated the defeminizing effects on lordosis behavior, but did not prevent anovulatory sterility (Table 7, Part 3; McEwen et al., 1977). CI-628 affords only partial protection against TP and produces a weak differential effect owing to its own weak estrogenicity (McEwen et al., 1977). That CI-628 may exert its effects by interfering with the action of estradiol derived from neural aromatization of T is supported by the work of Lieberburg and co-workers (1977b), who found that levels of $^3HE_2$

derived from an injection of ^{3}HT into 5-day-old female rats were reduced by prior administration of CI-628 on day 4 (Table 6). Tissue levels of $^3HE_2$ were unaltered by CI-628, suggesting that aromatization was unaffected. Likewise unaltered were tissue and cell nuclear levels of ^{3}HT and ^{3}HDHT.

In a bird species, the Japanese quail (Adkins, 1975), CI-628 is also reported to interfere with sexual differentiation in ovo, but the direction of the effects is opposite from that for mammals; namely, CI-628 blocks feminization of males by ovarian secretions. This pattern is consistent with other aspects of the pattern of sexual differentiation found among birds (see below).

It should be noted that the antiandrogen, cyproterone acetate, also inhibits androgenization (Arai and Gorski, 1968b). Although this observation would appear to contradict the success with antiestrogens, the antiandrogen may inhibit androgen action nonspecifically or by virtue of progestin action. Nevertheless, independent actions of androgens, as androgens and as estrogens after aromatization, have not been eliminated as possibilities. Recent work from the laboratory of Clemens and co-workers (1978; Gladue and Clemens, 1978) raises the possibility that androgen action before birth in the rat may involve androgen rather than estrogen receptors. In these studies, the antiandrogen, flutamide (4′-nitro-3′-trifluoromethylisobutyrylanilide), given to the mother during days 10 to 22 of gestation, was shown to attenuate both the development of masculine sexual behavior and the suppression of feminine sexual behavior in the rat. In the case of feminine sexual behavior, the main effect of flutamide treatment prenatally appears to be to enhance sensitivity of both male and female offspring to the lordosis-activating effects of estradiol. The mechanism of flutamide action is unknown at this time: blockade of androgen secretion, interference with androgen receptors, and even interference with aromatization and estrogen receptor function all remain as possibilities.

Fetoneonatal Estrogen-Binding Protein and Its Possible Protective Role in the Rat and Mouse

Fetal and neonatal rat blood contains, in abundance, an estrogen-binding protein (fEBP) produced by the yolk sac and embryonic liver (Nunez et al., 1971; Raynaud et al., 1971). This protein, which appears to be identical to α-fetoprotein (Uriel et al., 1972; Aussel et al., 1973), has a sedimentation coefficient in sucrose density gradients (SDG) of ~ 4S (Raynaud et al., 1971; Plapinger et al., 1973) and shows a marked preference for E_2 over synthetic estrogens, in contrast to the neonatal tissue receptor. Thus, whereas low doses of $^3HE_2$ are largely sequestered by fEBP and do not reach the cell nuclear receptor sites in significant amounts, comparable doses of the synthetic estrogen, ^{3}H-RU2858, do not bind to fEBP and do bind to brain cell nuclear receptor sites (Raynaud, 1973).

The fEBP is also found in cerebrospinal fluid and in washes of neonatal brain tissue and can, therefore, also be detected in cytosol from neonatal rat brains perfused at sacrifice to remove blood contamination (Plapinger et al., 1973). This protein reacts immunochemically like fEBP from blood (Plapinger and McEwen, 1975), and its presence in brain interferes with the detection of the true cytosol receptor sites unless one uses special methodological precautions with $^3HE_2$ as ligand (Barley et al., 1974) or uses a synthetic estrogen such as ^{3}H-RU2858. It remains to be determined whether the presence of fEBP in brains has any significance besides the protective function (Figure 29) ascribed to the blood fEBP (Soloff et al., 1971; Plapinger et al., 1973; Raynaud, 1973; Uriel and de Nechaud, 1973; McEwen et al., 1975). It is interesting to note, however, that mouse α-fetoprotein, believed to be identical to fEBP, binds to T lymphocytes (Dattwyler et al., 1975) and exerts an immunosuppressive action (Murgita and Tomasi, 1975). The involvement of E_2 in this action is unknown.

It may be predicted from the differential binding of $^3HE_2$ and ^{3}H-RU2858 by fEBP and by brain receptors that the latter would be more effective than E_2 in promoting sexual differentiation of the brain (Figure 29). Indeed, this appears to be the case, and dramatically so, from recent studies of Doughty and co-workers (1975a), showing a 50- to 100-fold difference in potency between RU2858 and E_2. RU-2858 is also more effective than E_2 in promoting uterine growth in rats during the first 2 weeks of postnatal life when titers of fEBP are high, and it is approximately equal to E_2 in effectiveness when fEBP titers are low or undetectable at the end of the third postnatal week of life (Raynaud et al., 1971). Diethylstilbestrol (DES), which is also a poor ligand for fEBP and which therefore binds better than E_2 to

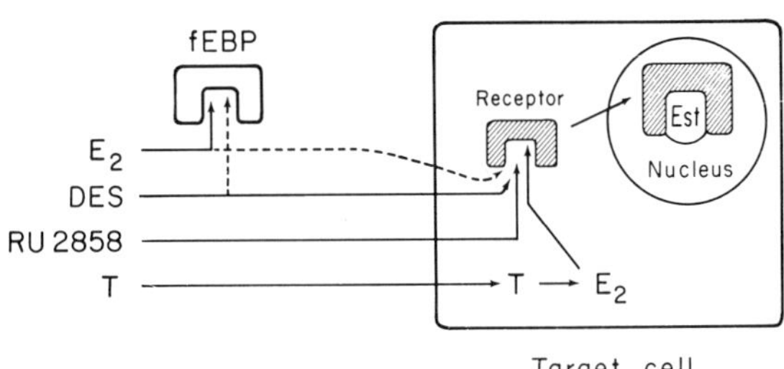

Figure 29. Schematic diagram of the protective role of fEBP and the ability of synthetic estrogens and testosterone to bypass this mechanism. E_2 = estradiol; DES = diethystilbestrol; RU2858 = 11β-methoxyethynylestradiol; T = testosterone; Est = various estrogens in the nucleus. [McEwen et al., 1975]

neonatal brain receptors, is also known to induce brain sexual differentiation at low doses (Kincl et al., 1965; Ladosky, 1967; Clemens, 1974).

Deleterious effects of estrogens are not confined to the brain; DES has been shown to induce reproductive tract abnormalities—masculine development of the reproductive tract and increased incident of primary vaginal carcinoma—in female human children exposed to DES in fetal life (Bongiovanni et al., 1959; Herbst et al., 1972). Yet the nature of protection of the human fetus from natural estrogens remains in question, as no one has established the existence of an estrogen-binding protein like α-fetoprotein in humans.

Estrogens, Aromatization, and Feminization of Bird Sexual Behavior

The role of estrogens in female sexual differentiation in birds has been highlighted by the recent work of Adkins (1975, 1976). The masculine or feminine status of adult Japanese quail was ascertained by noting behaviorally dimorphic sexual responses, which normally follow treatment with testosterone proprionate or estradiol benzoate. The sexual behavior of adult quail is sexually dimorphic. Males with circulating testosterone perform the sequence head grab-mount-cloacal contact movement, whereas females with circulating testosterone do not. When treated with exogenous estrogen as adults, the sexes do not differ in their capacity to display receptivity to a male attempting to copulate. Adkins suggests that embryonic estrogen results in female differentiation and produces the adult sex difference in mating behavior by eliminating the capacity for male sexual behavior in females. This interpretation is bolstered by three facts: (1) Female avian embryos produce significant quantities of estrogens (Ozon, 1965; Haffen, 1975); (2) the hypothalamus of the chick embryo appears to contain estrogen receptors and begins to retain labelled estradiol selectively prior to sex differentiation (Martinez-Vargas et al., 1975); and (3) Adkins' (1976) own observation that female Japanese quail exposed to the antiestrogen, CI-628, before hatching are "masculinized," as judged by their typically male adult response to TP treatment. Presumably, CI-628 prevents the embryo's own estrogen from exerting its feminizing (copulation-inhibiting) effect on the developing brain. However, a note of caution should be added here. Adult domestic fowl hens can become functional adult cocks and behave accordingly (Crew, 1923; Arnsdorf, 1947). Female-female pairing is relatively common among southern California's Western gulls. In such pairs one of the females may exhibit behaviors normally restricted to males, such as courtship feeding, mounting, and attempted copulation (Hunt and Hunt, 1977). Thus, it cannot be said that in all birds early exposure to estrogens eliminates the capacity for male sexual behavior in adulthood.

Gonadal Steroid Receptors in the Developing Mouse and Rat Brain

Estrogen and androgen receptors are present in the brain of the newborn rat and mouse. They appear each to be stereospecific for appropriate steroids and steroid antagonists and to resemble receptors found in adult brain, as well as in other endocrine target tissues. Their inferred action is to trigger changes in gene expression, which, in turn, influence the formation of synaptic connections through alterations in neurite outgrowth and other parameters discussed earlier in connection with morphological sex differences in the brain. And, as discussed in the previous section, there is now evidence that steroid receptors are at least partially occupied in males by estrogen derived from the aromatization of T and that aromatization is, in fact, one essential event for sexual differentiation of the rodent brain to occur.

Fox and colleagues have characterized putative androgen and estrogen receptors of the developing mouse brain (Fox and Johnston, 1974; Fox, 1975a,b; Wieland and Fox, 1976; Vito and Fox, 1977; Fox et al., 1978; Wieland et al., 1978). Using DNA-cellulose chromatography and SDG centrifugation, they initially examined cytosol receptors in 3-week-old mice. Hypothalamic-POA cytosol extracts, labeled with ^{3}H-E$_2$, showed macromolecular binding that adheres to DNA-cellulose and elutes at 210 mM NaCl, but does not adhere to cellulose columns alone (Figure 30A). This receptor sediments at 4S in SDG. If this receptor is heated to 30 to 37°C, then the receptor after elution from DNA sediments at 5S in SDG (Fox, 1977a). This is similar to uterine receptor forms, except that the uterine extract on DNA-celluose does not have to be heated for this conversion to the 5S "nuclear" form to occur.

Testosterone binds to macromolecules, of which the major fraction elutes from DNA-cellulose at 130 mM NaCl and a minor fraction at 210 mM NaCl (Figure 30B). DHT apparently binds to the same macromolecules (Wieland et al., 1978). Besides binding either to ^{3}H-testosterone or ^{3}H-dihydrotestosterone, the androgen binding by this presumed androgen receptor is substantially blocked by nonradioactive estradiol. There is a similar observation of estradiol blockade of androgen receptor from kidney (Bullock and Bardin, 1974).

That the androgen-binding component may truly be a receptor is indicated by its deficiency in the androgen-resistant mutant mouse (testicular feminization *Tfm*). The estradiol-binding level is normal in this mutant. The residual androgen binding in *Tfm* elutes at 210 mM NaCl (Figure 31). Fox is currently trying to determine whether it represents a low level of normal androgen receptor, a minor species that is normally present but is masked by a majority species, or a "mutant" macromolecule.

It is now evident that both androgen and estrogen receptors are present in the hypothalamus before birth (Fox et al., 1978; Maclusky et al., 1979; Vito and Fox, 1979). Quantitative demonstrations of estrogen receptors in the perinatal period require either their fractionation on DNA-cellulose to remove α-fetoprotein (Fox 1975a) or the use of ligands that are more selective for the receptor (McEwen et al., 1975). Developmental changes in levels of androgen and estrogen receptors appear to differ. In the mouse brain, for example, the relative increase of androgen receptors postnatally is greater than that of estrogen receptors (Attardi and Ohno, 1976). In the rat, however, the

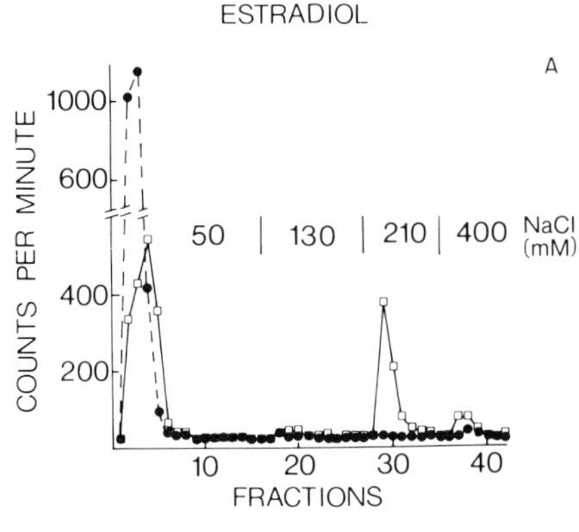

Figure 30. Chromatography of estrogen and androgen receptors on columns of DNA-cellulose (□) or cellulose (●). Extracts of the hypothalamus-preoptic area, labeled with either ^{3}H-estradiol (A) or ^{3}H-testosterone (B), were prepared from 3-week-old mice. [Wieland et al., 1978]

neural estrogen receptor levels increase sharply in the perinatal period, rising manyfold from 2 days before birth to a plateau around the end of the first postnatal week (Maclusky et al., 1979); so far, little is known about androgen receptor levels during this period. The sharp increase in estrogen receptors in the perinatal rat brain coincides with the onset of neural sensitivity to testosterone and estradiol as far as the postnatal suppression of ovulatory capability and feminine sexual behavior. This has prompted Maclusky and co-workers (1979) to suggest

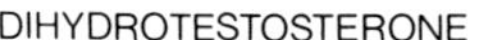

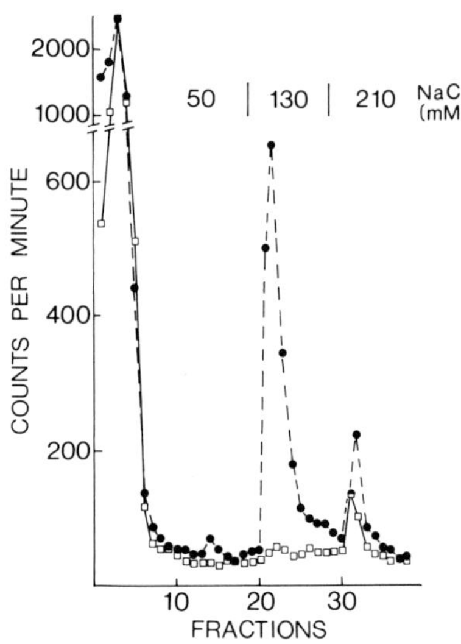

Figure 31. Comparison of putative androgen receptors from the hypothalamus-preoptic area of normal (•) and *Tfm*/T (□) mice by DNA-cellulose chromatography. [Wieland et al., 1978]

that the abrupt rise in estrogen receptors may be the event that determines the onset of this critical period, since it is known that both testosterone secretion and neural aromatizing enzyme activity are already established by this time. This possibility raises, in turn, a host of other largely unanswered questions. For example, what causes estrogen receptors to rise so sharply—another hormone, perhaps? And what aspect of hormonal sensitivity is involved in the developmental increase in masculine response potential, since this process appears largely separable from defeminization (see earlier discussion)? What about the prenatal period in view of the relative absence of estrogen receptors before fetal day 20 and in light of the work of the Clemens group showing effects of an antiandrogen flutamide during the prenatal period (see above)? Finally, what aspect of hormonal sensitivity and/or cell differentiation determines the end of the critical period? Fox proposed that it might somehow be a function of increasing androgen receptor levels in the first postnatal week of life. It also appears that maturational events, including synapse formation and myelinization, which are influenced by hormones like thyroxine, together with the increasing specialization of neuronal metabolism in this postnatal period, parallel the decreasing capacity of neurons for cell growth as well as the changing role of estrogen receptors from growth-related events à la Toran-Allerand to activational events related to neurotransmitter and energy metabolism.

V. CELLULAR BASES OF SEXUAL DIMORPHISMS OF BRAIN STRUCTURE AND FUNCTION

The Work Session began with a definition of "sexually dimorphic behaviors" and introduced the concept of the organization of such behaviors during a critical period of development. Such critical periods are known to exist for birds and mammals. Their existence in lower vertebrate forms has not been clearly established, and so it is impossible to say at this time whether there are systematic phylogenetic differences in the occurrence of this important phenomenon. For mammals and birds, the organization of sexually dimorphic behaviors appears to involve permanent changes in brain structure and function during a time when many neurons are extending processes and forming synapses. For the most part, these changes are attributable to the actions of gonadal steroids elaborated primarily in one sex during the critical period. These steroids act on a bipotential reproductive tract and brain to cause the expression or accentuation of a genetic program specific for the individual, strain, and species (Figure 32). It is important to stress this last point, since the organizational effects of the gonadal hormones on certain traits are somewhat analogous to the actions of a photographic developer to call forth a latent image. A case in point is the effect of neonatal androgen in calling forth strain-typical levels of aggressive behavior in females of three mouse strains (Vale et al., 1972).

Figure 32 emphasizes that the genome programs the following three properties: (1) the sex of the gonad, (2) the elaboration of enzymes and receptors that constitute the hormone response system of

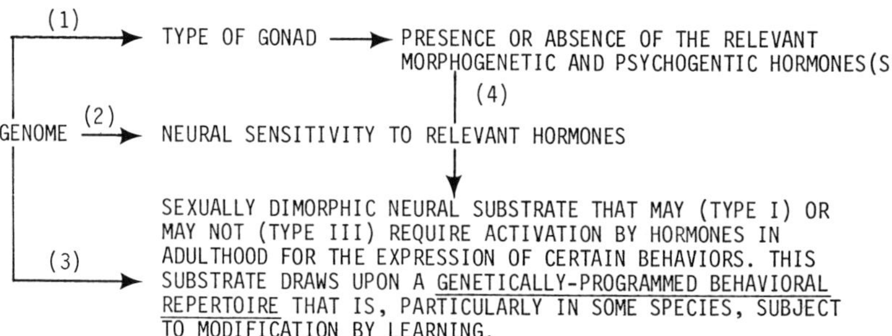

Figure 32. Role of genetic factors in sexual differentiation. [McEwen]

the developing brain, and (3) the behavioral repertoire. As noted in this report of the Work Session, loss of the Y chromosome upsets (1) and results in Turner's syndrome, in which gonadal tissue is virtually absent, whereas genetic changes less drastic than chromosomal loss can result in abnormalities in the hormone response system represented by (2) and lead, for instance, to the various forms of androgen insensitivity, which, in turn, may influence the process of sexual differentiation as well as adult neuroendocrine function. Variability of the genetic factors that constitute the third contribution of the genome ((3) in Figure 32) crops up as species differences in the behavioral repertoire, or as the subtler consequences of chromosomal reassortment in crosses between two strains of the same species (e.g., the appearance of reduced androgen dependence of male sexual behavior in the BD_2F_1 mouse strain).

A major goal of the Work Session was to understand better the sequence of events in the developing brain that gives rise to sexually dimorphic behaviors. Before considering these events, we must first consider the state of the brain at the time they occur: whether the responsive cells are still capable of undergoing cell divisions as well as other aspects of their state of differentiation pertaining to hormonal sensitivity. The rodent brain has been studied in sufficient depth to provide such insights, and we know for the rat that neurons of two of the most important brain regions, the preoptic area and hypothalamus, have undergone final cell divisions (Ifft, 1972) by the time of the first testicular activity on fetal day 16. We also know that aromatizing enzyme activity appears at about the same time as testicular activity, but that estrogen receptors increase markedly several days later, shortly before birth on day 22. Thus, with respect to the aspects of brain sexual differentiation in the rat, which are dependent on aromatization of testosterone as well as estrogen receptors (i.e., defeminization of feminine sexual behavior and ovulatory potential), the appearance of estrogen receptors (e.g., item (4) in Figure 32) may be the critical event determining the onset of the process. As noted in this volume, the differentiation of the capacity for male sexual behavior is a separate process that begins before birth in the rat and may not depend exclusively on aromatization but rather on androgens and androgen receptors. We still have no idea what factors cause the appropriate brain cells to express their genetic program for steroid metabolizing enzymes and steroid receptors; whatever they are, these factors do appear to operate in both sexes, for the brains of both female and male rats respond to testosterone present during the critical period.

The Work Session provided new information regarding sex differences in brain structure, which appear to arise as a result of the action of gonadal steroids during the critical period (item (4) in Figure 32) in both birds and mammals. Since these morphological features involve at least three aspects of brain structure (i.e., the type of synapse, the shape of the dendritic tree, and the size of a group of cells known as a nucleus to neuroanatomists), one wonders whether there is a single or multiple explanation for their origin(s). One attractive, unifying explanation for morphological sex differences derives from the work of Toran-Allerand (see above) on steroid-induced outgrowth of neurites from hypothalamic and preoptic area explants of newborn mice. Were such changes to take place in the intact male brain as a result of perinatal testicular secretion, the more rapid growth of neurites might well permit the development of different as well as more numerous synaptic connections and lead to alterations of the final shape of the dendritic tree.

There are two possible reasons for differences in the size of a group of cells, as described for the rat by Gorski and for the songbird by Nottebohm, namely, cell number or individual cell size and packing arrangement. If it is cell size that is involved, then how does this relate to neurite outgrowth? One attractive possibility is that larger cell bodies may be ones that have established larger terminal projection fields and/or larger dendritic trees. With respect to the possibility of differences in cell number, the lack of cell divisions among the responsive neurons of the hypothalamus and preoptic area at the time of sexual differentiation (Ifft, 1972) means that any difference in cell number would have to result from steroid-induced cell destruction or survival. This could come about either as a direct result of steroid action, unrelated to neurite outgrowth, or it might be the result of neurite outgrowth and synapse formation. This latter statement is based on the well-organized principle of neural development: neurons that fail to establish sufficient numbers of synapses with permissible cells tend to die and disappear (Prestige, 1970; Landmesser and Pilar, 1978).

Having in mind an explanation of brain sexual differentiation based on differential neuronal growth under hormonal control, we shall return to our attempts to find generalizations across vertebrate species. For reasons stated in the first paragraph, we shall speak only of birds and mammals. Two questions are of great interest: The first is the nature of the hormonal signal. In birds, it is an ovarian product, probably estradiol; in mammals it is a testicular product, testosterone. In some but not all mammals, estradiol, arising from testosterone by local metabolism in the brain, is an essential part of brain sexual differentiation. Yet in guinea pigs and in primates (including man), androgens and androgen receptors appear to be of greater importance than estrogens in brain sexual differentiation. Aside from the disappointment of not finding a single hormonal agent responsible for brain sexual differentiation in birds and mammals, there is nothing in the model of neurite outgrowth presented for the rat and mouse that is incompatible with an androgen-receptor-mediated neurite outgrowth in target neurons of fetal guinea pig and primate brains. The second question is whether there are morphological sex differences in brains of mammals other than rodents. We still do not have information to answer this question. However, in view of similarities in the distribution of steroid hormone receptors and steroid-metabolizing enzymes in rodent and primate brains (e.g., see Morrell et al., 1975; Naftolin et al., 1975b), and because of similarities in other aspects of brain structure and neuroendocrine function among all mammals, it is a good bet that such morphological sex differences are also widespread among mammals. The same view might be advanced regarding the possible generalization from songbirds to other birds, although morphological sex differences need not exist in the same brain regions of all bird species.

Even if morphological sex differences do exist in the human brain more or less as they occur in the rat brain, we must deal with another important issue that was repeatedly expressed at the Work Session; namely, the relatively greater influence in our own species of social factors and learning in sex differences in behavior. Even gender role behavior, which is subject to prenatal androgen influences and in this respect is at least analogous to sexually differentiated behaviors in rats, develops under the strong influence of learning acting upon an endocrinologically biased substrate. The task of discerning an endocrine component, as opposed to influences of learning, in sexual orientation (see discussion of homosexuality) appears to be even more difficult than that of detecting an endocrine influence on gender role behavior. There is a need to ask why a hormonal influence on sexual orientation is so difficult to discern in human beings. Is it because the endocrine influence is nonexistent or weak relative to social conditioning? Is it because the human genome accommodates a high degree of bisexuality, or at least bisexual potential, in each of us? Or is it because the individual who might be prone to discordant sexual orientation finds it easier to learn to act out the proscribed role than to defy societal mores and parental expectations and to violate strongly established taboos? From our discussions, the biological substrate seems important in the human being as in other mammals, and one of the contributions of the Work Session may have been to give this aspect of sexual differentiation a full hearing.

ABBREVIATIONS

ADX	adrenalectomized
AHA	anterior hypothalamic area
AI	androgen insensitivity
ATD	androst-1,4,6-triene-3,17-dione
CAH	congenital adrenal hyperplasia
DAS	delayed anovulatory syndrome
DES	diethylstilbestrol
DHT	5α-dihydrotestosterone
DHTP	dihydrotestosterone propionate
DRL	differential reinforcement of low rates of response
E_2	17β-estradiol
EB	estradiol benzoate
FALE	feminine males
fEBP	fetoneonatal estrogen-binding protein
FSH	follicle-stimulating hormone
HVc	hyperstriatum ventrale, pars caudale
LH	luteinizing hormone
LHRH	luteinizing hormone-releasing hormone
pc	postconception
POA	preoptic area
RA	robust nucleus of the archistriatum
SCN	suprachiasmatic nucleus
SDG	sucrose density gradient
T	testosterone
TG	testosterone glucuronide
TP	testosterone propionate
VMH	ventromedial hypothalamus

BIBLIOGRAPHY

This bibliography contains two types of entries: (1) citations given or work alluded to in the report, and (2) additional references to pertinent literature by conference participants and others.

Abramovich, D.R. and Rowe, P. (1973): Foetal plasma testosterone levels at mid-pregnancy and at term: relationship to fetal sex. *J. Endocrinol.* 56:621-622.

Adams-Smith, W.N. (1970): Transplacental influence of androgen upon ovulatory mechanisms in the rat. *J. Endocrinol.* 48: 477-478.

Adkins, E.K. (1975): Hormonal basis of sexual differentiation in the Japanese quail. *J. Comp. Physiol. Psychol.* 89:61-71.

Adkins, E.K. (1976): Embryonic exposure to an antiestrogen masculinizes behavior of female quail. *Physiol. Behav.* 17:357-359.

Adkins, E.K. (1977): Effects of diverse androgens on the sexual behavior and morphology of castrated male quail. *Horm. Behav.* 8:201-207.

Alsum, P. and Goy, R.W. (1974): Actions of esters of testosterone, dihydrotestosterone, or estradiol on sexual behavior in castrated male guinea pigs. *Horm. Behav.* 5:207-217.

Anderson, C.O. (1970): Maternal behavior in the rabbit. *Horm. Behav.* 1:337-345.

Anderson, J.N., Peck, J.R., and Clark, J.H. (1975): Estrogen-induced uterine responses and growth: relationship to receptor estrogen binding by uterine nuclei. *Endocrinology* 96:160-167.

Anisko, J.J., Christenson, T., and Buehler, M.G. (1973): Effects of androgen on fighting behavior in male and female Mongolian gerbils, *Meriones unguiculatus. Horm. Behav.* 4:199-208.

Aono, T., Miyake, A., Kinugasa, T., Kurachi, K., and Matsumoto, K. (1978): Absence of positive feedback effect of oestrogen on LH release in patients with testicular feminization syndrome. *Acta Endocrinol.* 87:259-267.

Arai, Y. and Gorski, R.A. (1968a): The critical exposure time for androgenization of the developing hypothalamus in the female rat. *Endocrinology* 82:1010-1014.

Arai, Y. and Gorski, R.A. (1968b): Critical exposure time for androgenization of the rat hypothalamus determined by anti-androgen injection. *Proc. Soc. Exp. Biol. Med.* 127:590-593.

Arai, Y. and Gorski, R.A. (1968c): Protection against the neural organizing effect of exogenous androgen in the neonatal female rat. *Endocrinology* 82:1005-1009.

Arai, Y. and Gorski, R.A. (1974): Possible participation of pituitary testicular feedback regulation in the sexual differentiation of the brain in the male rat. *In: Biological Rhythms in Neuroendocrine Activity.* Kawakami, M., ed. Tokyo: Igaku Shoin, Ltd., pp. 232-240.

Araki, S., Toran-Allerand, D., Ferin, M., and Vande Wiele, R.L. (1975): Immunoreactive gonadotrophin releasing hormone during maturation in the rat: Ontogeny of regional hypothalamic differences. *Endocrinology* 97:693-697.

Archer, J. (1975): Rodent sex differences in emotional and related behavior. *Behav. Biol.* 14:451-479.

Arms, S. (1975): *Immaculate Deception: A New Look at Women and Childbirth in America.* Boston: Houghton Mifflin.

Armstrong, E.A. (1955): *The Wren.* London: Collins.

Armstrong, E.A. (1963): *A Study of Bird Song.* London: Oxford University Press.

Arnold, A.P. (1974): Behavioral effects of androgen in zebra finches *(Poephila guttata)* and a search for its sites of action. Ph.D. Dissertation, Rockefeller University, New York.

Arnold, A.P. (1975a): The effects of castration and androgen replacement on song, courtship, and aggression in zebra finches *(Poephila guttata). J. Exp. Zool.* 191:309-326.

Arnold, A.P. (1975b): The effects of castration on song development in zebra finches *(Poephila guttata). J. Exp. Zool.* 191:261-278.

Arnold, A.P., Nottebohm, F., and Pfaff, D.W. (1976): Hormone concentrating cells in vocal control and other areas of the brain of the zebra finch *(Poephila guttata). J. Comp. Neurol.* 165:487-512.

Arnsdorf, R.E. (1947): Hen into rooster. *J. Hered.* 38:320.

Attardi, B., Geller, L., and Ohno, S. (1976): Androgen and estrogen receptors in brain cytosol from male, female, and testicular feminized (tfm/y) hermaphrodite mice. *Endocrinology* 98:864-874.

Attardi, B. and Ohno, S. (1976): Androgen and estrogen receptors in the developing mouse brain. *Endocrinology* 99:1279-1290.

Aussel, C., Uriel, J., and Mercier-Bodard, C. (1973): Rat alpha-fetoprotein: isolation, characterization and estrogen-binding properties. *Biochimie* 55:1431-1437.

Bailey, D.W. (1971): Recombinant-inbred strains. *Transplantation* 11:325-327.

Baker, S.W. and Ehrhardt, A.A. (1974): Prenatal androgens, intelligence and cognitive sex differences. *In: Sex Differences in Behavior.* Friedman, R.C., Richart, R.M., and Vande Wiele, R.L., eds. New York: John Wiley and Sons, Inc., pp. 33-51.

Baldwin, F.M., Goldin, H.S., and Metfessel, M. (1940): Effects of testosterone propionate on female roller canaries under complete song isolation. *Proc. Soc. Exp. Biol. Med.* 44:373-375.

Barfield, R.J. and Geyer, L.A. (1975): The ultrasonic post-ejaculatory vocalization and the post-ejaculatory refractory period of the male rat. *J. Comp. Physiol. Psychol.* 88:723-734.

Barley, J., Ginsburg, M., Greenstein, B.D., MacLusky, N.J., and Thomas, P.J. (1974): A receptor mediating sexual differentiation? *Nature* 252:259-260.

Barlow, G.W. (1977): Modal action patterns. *In: How Animals Communicate.* Sebeok, T.A., ed. Bloomington, Ind.: University of Indiana Press, pp. 98-134.

Barnea, A. and Lindner, H.R. (1972): Short-term inhibition of macromolecular synthesis and androgen-induced sexual differentiation of the rat brain. *Brain Res.* 45:479-487.

Barraclough, C.A. (1966): Modifications in the CNS regulation of reproduction after exposure of prepubertal rats to steroid hormones. *Rec. Prog. Horm. Res.* 22:503-539.

Barraclough, C.A. and Gorski, R.A. (1962): Studies on mating behavior in the androgen-sterilized rat and their relation to the hypothalamic regulation of sexual behavior in the female rat. *J.Endocrinol.* 25:175-182.

Barraclough, C.A. and Leathem, J.H. (1954): Infertility induced in mice by a single injection of testosterone propionate. *Proc. Soc. Exp. Biol. Med.* 85:673-674.

Barrett, R.J. and Ray, O.S. (1970): Behavior in the open field, Lashley III maze, shuttle-box, and Sidman avoidance as a function of strain, sex and age. *Dev. Psychol.* 3:73-77.

Baum, M.J. (1976): Effects of testosterone propionate administered perinatally on sexual behavior of female ferrets. *J. Comp. Physiol. Psychol.* 90:399-410.

Baum, M.J. and Schretlen, P. (1975): Neuroendocrine effects of perinatal androgenization in the male ferret. *Prog. Brain Res.* 42:343-355.

Baum, M.J., Södersten, P., and Vreeburg, J.T.M. (1974): Mounting and receptive behavior in the ovariectomized female rat: Influence of estradiol, dihydrotestoterone, and genital anaesthetization. *Horm. Behav.* 5:175-190.

Baum, M.J. and Vreeburg, J.T.M. (1973): Copulation in castrated male rats following combined treatment with estradiol and dihydrotesterone. *Science* 182:283-285.

Beach, F.A. (1961): *Hormones and Behavior.* 2nd Ed. New York: Cooper Square.

Beach, F.A. (1971): Hormonal factors controlling the differentiation, development, and display of copulatory behavior in the ramstergig and related species. *In: The Biopsychology of Development.* Tobach, E., Aronson, L.R., and Shaw, E., eds. New York: Academic Press, pp. 249-296.

Beach, F.A. (1974): Effects of gonadal hormones in urinary behavior in dogs. *Physiol. Behav.* 12:1005-1013.

Beach, F.A. (1976): Sexual attractivity, proceptivity and receptivity in female mammals. *Horm. Behav.* 7:105-138.

Beach, F.A. and Buehler, M.G. (1977): Male rats with inherited insensitivity to androgen show reduced sexual behavior. *Endocrinology* 100:197-200.

Beach, F.A. and Kuehn, R.E. (1970): Coital behavior in dogs. X. Effects of androgenic stimulation during development on feminine mating responses in females and males. *Horm. Behav.* 1:347-367.

Beach, F.A., Kuehn, R.E., Sprague, R.H., and Anisko, J.J. (1972): Coital behavior in dogs. XI. Effects of androgenic stimulation during development on masculine mating responses in females. *Horm. Behav.* 3:143-168.

Beatty, W.W. (1973a): Effects of gonadectomy on sex differences in DRL behavior. *Physiol. Behav.* 10:177-178.

Beatty, W.W. (1973b): Postneonatal testosterone treatment fails to alter hormonal regulation of body weight and food intake of female rats. *Physiol. Behav.* 10:627-628.

Beatty, W.W. (1977): Sex differences in DRL and active avoidance behaviors in the rat depend upon the day-night cycle. *Bull. Psychon. Soc.* 10:95-97.

Beatty, W.W. and Beatty, P.A. (1970): Hormonal determinants of sex differences in avoidance behavior and reactivity to electric shock in the rat. *J. Comp. Physiol. Psychol.* 73:446-455.

Beatty, W.W., Bierley, C.M., and Gerth, J.G. (1975a): Effects of neonatal gonadectomy on DRL behavior. *Bull. Psychon. Soc.* 6:615.

Beatty, W.W. and Fessler, R.G. (1977a): Gonadectomy and sensitivity to electric shock in the rat. *Physiol. Behav.* 19:1-6.

Beatty, W.W. and Fessler, R.G. (1977b). Sex differences in sensitivity to electric shock in rats and hamsters. *Bull. Psychon. Soc.* 10:189-190.

Beatty, W.W., Gregoire, K.C., and Parmiter, L.L. (1973): Sex differences in retention of passive avoidance behavior in rats. *Bull. Psychon.* Soc. 2:99-100.

Beatty, W.W., O'Briant, D.A., and Vilberg, T.R. (1975b): Effects of ovariectomy and estradiol injections on food intake and body weight in rats with ventromedial hypothalamic lesions. *Pharmacol. Biochem. Behav.* 3:539-544.

Beatty, W.W., Powley, T.L., and Keesey, R.E. (1970): Effects of neonatal testosterone injection and hormone replacement in adulthood on body weight and body fat in female rats. *Physiol. Behav.* 5:1093-1098.

Beatty, W.W. and Siders, W.A. (1977): Effects of small lesions in the globus pallidus on open field and avoidance behavior in male and female rats. *Bull. Psychon. Soc.* 10:98-100.

Beckwith, B.E., Sandman, C.A., Hothersall, D., and Kastin, A.J. (1977): Influence of neonatal injections of α MSH on learning, memory and attention in rats. *Physiol. Behav.* 18:63-71.

Beeman, E.A. (1947): The effect of male hormone on aggressive behavior in mice. *Physiol. Zool.* 20:373-405.

Belisle, S., Fencl, M.M., and Tulchinsky, D. (1977): Amniotic fluid testosterone and follicle-stimulating hormone in the determination of fetal sex. *Am. J. Obstet. Gynecol.* 128:514-519.

Bell, D.D. and Zucker, I. (1971): Sex differences in body weight and eating: Organization and activation by gonadal hormones in the rat. *Physiol. Behav.* 7:27-34.

Bengelloun, W.A., Nelson, D.J., Zent, H.M., and Beatty, W.W. (1976): Behavior of male and female rats with septal lesions: Influence of prior gonadectomy. *Physiol. Behav.* 16:317-330.

Bennet-Clark, H.C., Ewing, A.W., and Manning, A. (1973): The persistence of courtship stimulation in *Drosophila melanogaster. Behav. Biol.* 8:763-769.

Benno, R.H. and Williams, T.H. (1977): Intracellular localization of alpha-fetoprotein (αFP) in the developing rat brain – an immunocytochemical study. *In: Society for Neuroscience Abstracts, Vol. III.* (Seventh Annual Meeting of the Society for Neuroscience, Anaheim, CA, Nov. 6-10, 1977.) P. 100.

Benoit, J. (1923): Transformation expérimentale du sexe par ovariotomie précoce chez la poule domestique. *C.R. Acad. Sci. B* 177:1074-1077.

Benoit, J. (1936): Stimulation par la lumière de l'activité sexuelle chez le canard et la cane domestiques. *Bull. Biol. Fr. Belg.* 70:487-533.

Berger, B., Hackette, B., and Miller, R.M. (1972): The communal family. *The Family Coordinator* 21:419-428.

Bernard, B.K. and Paolino, R.M. (1975): Temporal effects of castration on emotionality and shock-induced aggression in adult male rats. *Physiol. Behav.* 14:201-206.

Bernstein, I.S. and Sharpe, L.G. (1966): Social roles in a rhesus monkey group. *Behaviour* 36:91-104.

Bertram, B. (1970): The vocal behavior of the Indian hill mynah, *Gracula religiosa. Anim. Behav.* 3:81-192.

Beyer, C., de la Torre, L., Larsson, K., and Perez-Palacios, G. (1975): Synergistic actions of estrogen and androgen on the sexual behavior of the castrated male rabbit. *Horm. Behav.* 6:301-306.

Beyer, C. and Rivaud, N. (1973): Differential effect of testosterone and dihydrotestosterone on the sexual behavior of prepuberally castrated male rabbits. *Horm. Behav.* 4:175-180.

Beyer, C. and Vidal, N. (1971): Inhibitory action of MER-25 on androgen-induced oestrous behavior in the ovariectomized rabbit. *J. Endocrinol.* 51:401-402.

Bielert, C. (1978): Androgen treatments of young male rhesus monkeys, *In: Recent Advances in Primatology, Vol. I. Behaviour.* Chivers, D.J. and Herbert, J., eds. London: Academic Press, pp. 485-488.

Black, V.H. and Christensen, A.K. (1969): Differentiation of interstitial cells and Sertoli cells in fetal guinea pig testes. *Am. J. Anat.* 124:211-237.

Blizard, D. and Denef, C. (1973): Neonatal androgen effects on open-field activity and sexual behavior in the female rat: the modifying influence of ovarian secretions during development. *Physiol. Behav.* 11:65-69.

Blizard, D.A., Lippman, H.R., and Chen, J.J. (1975): Sex differences in open-field behavior in the rat: The inductive and activational role of gonadal hormones. *Physiol. Behav.* 14:601-608.

Bloch, E., Gupta, C., Feldman, S., and Van Damme, O. (1975): Testosterone production by testes of fetal rats and mice. *In: Endocrinologie Sexuelle de la Période Périnatal.* Paris: *INSERM* 32:177-189.

Blurton-Jones, N.G., ed. (1972): *Ethological Studies of Child Behaviour.* Cambridge: Cambridge University Press.

Bongiovanni, A.M., DiGeorge, A.M., and Grumbach, M.M. (1959): Masculinization of the female infant associated with estrogen therapy alone during gestation: four cases. *J. Clin. Endocrinol. Metab.* 19:1004-1011.

Booth, J.E. (1977a): Effects of the aromatization inhibitor, androst-4-ene-3,6,17-trione on sexual differentiation induced by testosterone in the neonatally castrated rat. *J. Endocrinol.* 72:53P-54P.

Booth, J.E. (1977b): Sexual behavior of neonatally castrated rats injected during infancy with oestrogen and dihydrotestosterone. *J. Endocrinol.* 72:135-141.

Boss, W.R. and Witschi, E. (1947): The permanent effect of early stilbestrol injections on the sex organs of the herring gull (*Larus argentatus*). *J. Exp. Zool.* 105:61-77.

Breuer, H. and Köster, G. (1975): Interaction between estrogens and neurotransmitters. Biochemical mechanism. *Adv. Biosci.* 15:287-300.

Brinkman, A.O. (1977): Testosterone synthesis *in vitro* by the fetal testis of the guinea pig. *Steroids* 29:861-873.

Bronson, F.H. and Desjardins, C.H. (1968): Aggression in adult mice: Modification by neonatal injections of gonadal hormones. *Science* 161:705-706.

Bronson, F.H. and Desjardins, C. (1970): Neonatal androgen administration and adult aggressiveness in female mice. *Gen. Comp. Endocrinol.* 15:320-325.

Bronstein, P.M. and Hirsch, S.M. (1974): Reactivity in the rat: Ovariectomy fails to affect open-field behaviors. *Bull. Psychon. Soc.* 3:257-260.

Brown-Grant, K. (1973): Recent studies on sexual differentiation of the brain. *In: Foetal and Neonatal Physiology.* Comline, K.S., et al., eds. New York: Cambridge University Press, pp. 527-545.

Brown-Grant, K. (1974): Failure of ovulation after administration of steroid hormones and hormone antagonists to female rats during the neonatal period. *J. Endocrinol.* 62:683-684.

Brown-Grant, K. (1975): A re-examination of the lordosis response in female rats given high doses of testosterone propionate or estradiol benzoate in the neonatal period. *Horm. Behav.* 6:351-378.

Brown-Grant, K., Fink, G., Greig, F., and Murray, M. (1975): Altered sexual development in male rats after oestrogen administration during the neonatal period. *J. Reprod. Fertil.* 44:25-42.

Brown-Grant, K. and Sherwood, M.R. (1971): The "early androgen syndrome" in the guinea pig. *J. Endrocrinol.* 49:277-291.

Buchanan, O.M. (1966): Homosexual behavior in wild orange-fronted parakeets. *Condor* 68:399-400.

Bullock, L.P. and Bardin, C.W. (1974): Androgen receptors in mouse kidney: a study of male, female and androgen-insensitive (tfm/y) mice. *Endocrinology* 94:746-755.

Bullock, L.P., Mainwaring, W.I.P., and Bardin, C.W. (1975): The physicochemical properties of the cytoplasmic androgen receptor in the kidneys of normal carrier female (tfm/+) and androgen-insensitive (tfm/y) mice. *Endocrinol. Res. Commun.* 2:25-45.

Burns, R.K. (1961): Role of hormones in the differentiation of sex. *In: Sex and Internal Secretions.* Young, W.C., ed. Baltimore: Williams and Wilkins, pp. 76-158.

Campbell, A.B. and McGill, T.E. (1970): Neonatal hormone treatment and sexual behavior in male mice. *Horm. Behav.* 1:145-150.

Campbell, H.J. (1965): Effects of neonatal injections of hormones in sexual behavior and reproduction in the rabbit. *J. Physiol.* 181:568-575.

Carpenter, C.R. (1942): Societies of monkeys and apes. *Biol. Symp.* 8:177-204. Reprinted *In: Primate Social Behavior.* Southwick, C.H., ed. (1963): Princeton, NJ: D. Van Nostrand, Inc., pp. 24-51.

Carter, C.S., Clemens, L.G., and Hoekema, D.J. (1972): Neonatal androgen and adult sexual behavior in the golden hamster. *Physiol. Behav.* 9:89-95.

Carter, C.S. and Landauer, M.R. (1975): Neonatal hormone experience and adult lordosis and fighting in the golden hamster. *Physiol. Behav.* 14:1-6.

Cavazza, F. (1938): Ricerche sperimentali sui caratteri sessuali secondari ed il dimorfismo stagionale di *Anas boscas* L. *Arch. Zool. Exp. Gen.* 79:409-461.

Challis, J.R.G., Kim, C.K., Naftolin, F., Judd, H.L., Yen, S.S.C., and Bernirschke, K. (1974): The concentrations of androgens, oestrogens, progesterone and luteinizing hormone in the serum of foetal calves throughout the course of gestation. *J. Endocrinol.* 60:107-115.

Chambers, K.C. (1976): Hormonal influence on sexual dimorphism in rate of extinction of a conditioned taste aversion in rats. *J. Comp. Physiol. Phychol.* 90:851-856.

Charnov, E.L. and Bull, J. (1977): When is sex environmentally determined? *Nature* 266:828-830.

Cheng, M-F. and Lehrman, D. (1975): Gonadal hormone specificity in the sexual behavior of ring doves. *Psychoneuroendocrinology* 1:95-102.

Choat, H.G. and Robertson, D.R. (1975): Protogynous hermaphroditism in fishes of the family *Scaridae. In: Intersexuality in the Animal Kingdom.* Reinboth. R., ed. New York: Springer-Verlag, pp. 263-283.

Choudhury, M. and Steinberger, E. (1976): Pituitary and plasma levels of gonadotrophins in foetal and newborn male and female rats. *J. Endocrinol.* 69:381-384.

Christensen, L.W., Coniglio, L.P., Paup, D.C., and Clemens, L.G. (1973): Sexual behavior of male golden hamsters receiving diverse androgen treatments. *Horm. Behav.* 4:223-229.

Christensen, L.W. and Gorski, R.A. (1978): Independent masculinization of neuroendocine systems by intracerebral implants of testosterone or estradiol in the neonatal female rat. *Brain Res.* 146:325-340

Christensen, L.W., Nance, D.M., and Gorski, R.A. (1977): Effects of hypothalamic and preoptic lesions on reproductive behavior in male rats. *Brain Res. Bull.* 2:137-141.

Christenson, T., Wallen, K., Brown, B.A., and Glickman, S.E. (1973): Effects of castration, blindness, and anosmia on social reactivity in the male Mongolian gerbil, *Meriones unguiculatus. Physiol. Behav.* 10:989-994.

Clark, J.H., Raszko, Z., and Peck, E.J., Jr. (1977): Nuclear binding and retention of the receptor estrogen complex: relation to agonistic and antagonistic properties of estriol. *Endocrinology* 100:91-96.

Clarke, I.J., Scaramuzzi, R.J., and Short, R.V. (1976a): The effect of testosterone implants in pregnant ewes on their female offspring. *J. Embryol. Exp. Morphol.* 36:87-99.

Clarke, I.J., Scaramuzzi, R.J., and Short, R.V. (1976b). Sexual differentiation of the brain: endocrine and behavioral responses of androgenized ewes to oestrogen. *J. Endocrinol.* 71:175-176.

Clarke, I.J., Scaramuzzi, R.J., and Short, R.V. (1977): Ovulation in prenatally androgenized ewes. *J. Endocrinol.* 75:385-389.

Clayton, R.B., Kogura, J., and Kraemer, H.C. (1970): Sexual differentiation of the brain: Effects of testosterone in brain RNA metabolism in newborn female rats. *Nature* 226: 810-812.

Clemens, H.P. and Inslee, T. (1968): The production of unisexual broods of *Tilapia mossambica* sex-reversed with methyltestosterone. *Trans. Am. Fish Soc.* 97:18-21.

Clemens, L.G. (1974): Neurohormonal control of male sexual behavior. *In: Reproductive Behavior.* Montagna, W. and Sadler, W.A., eds. New York: Plenum Press, pp. 23-53.

Clemens, L.G. and Coniglio, L. (1971): Influence of prenatal litter composition on mounting behavior of female rats. *Am. Zool.* 11:617-618. (Abstr.)

Clemens, L.G., Gladue, B.A., and Coniglio, L.P. (1978): Prenatal endogenous androgenic influences on masculine sexual behavior and genital morphology in male and female rats. *Horm. Behav.* 10:40-53.

Clemens, L.G., Hiroi, M., and Gorski, R.A. (1969): Induction and facilitation of female mating behavior in rats treated neonatally with low doses of testosterone propionate. *Endocrinology* 84:1430-1438.

Clemens, L.G., Shryne, J., and Gorski, R.A. (1970): Androgen and development of progesterone responsiveness in male and female rats. *Physiol. Behav.* 5:673-678.

Clements, J.A., Reyes, F.I., Winter, J.S.D., and Faiman, C. (1976): Studies on human sexual development. III. Fetal pituitary and serum, and amniotic fluid concentrations of LH, CG, and FSH. *Clin. Endocrinol. Metab.* 42:9-19.

Cochran, C.A. and Perachio, A.A. (1977): Dihydrotestosterone propionate effects on dominance and sexual behaviors in gonadectomized male and female rhesus monkeys. *Horm. Behav.* 8:175-187.

Collard, J. and Grevendal, L. (1946): L'étude sur les caractères sexueles des pinsons, *Fringilla coelebs* L. et *Fringilla montifringilla* L. *Gerfaut Rev. Sci. Belge Ornithol.* 36:89-107.

Collias, E.C. and Collias, N.E., (1973): Further studies on development of nest-building behaviour in a weavebird (*Ploceus cucullatus*). *Anim. Behav.* 21:371-382.

Collias, N.E. and Collias, E.C. (1962): An experimental study of the mechanisms of nest building in a weaverbird. *Auk* 79:568-595.

Collias, N.E. and Collias, E.C. (1967): A quantitative analysis of breeding behavior in the African village weaverbird. *Auk* 84:396-411.

Colvin, G.B. and Sawyer, C.H. (1969): Induction of running activity by intracerebral implants of estrogen in ovariectomized rats. *Neuroendocrinology* 4:309-320.

Coniglio, L.P., Paup, D.C., and Clemens, L.G. (1973): Hormonal factors controlling the development of sexual behavior in the male golden hamster. *Physiol. Behav.* 10:1087-1096.

Coniglio, L.P., Paup, D.C., and Clemens, L.G. (1973): Hormonal specificity in the suppression of sexual receptivity of the female golden hamster. *J. Endocrinol.* 57:55-61.

Conner, R.L., Levine, S., Wertheim, G.A., and Cummer, J.F. (1969): Hormonal determinants of aggressive behavior. *Ann. N.Y. Acad. Sci.* 159:760-776.

Corey, S.M. (1930): Sex differences in maze learning by white rats. *J. Comp. Psychol.* 10:333-338.

Count, E.W. (1973): *Being and Becoming Human: Essays on the Biogram.* New York: Van Nostrand Reinhold.

Crew, F.A.E. (1923): Sex reversal in the fowl. *Proc. Roy. Soc. B* 95:256-278.

Crowley, W.R., O'Donohue, T.L., and Jacobowitz, D.M. (1977): Gonadal hormone-catecholamine interactions in discrete regions of the central nervous system. *In: Neuroscience Abstracts, Vol. III.* (Seventh Annual Meeting of the Society for Neuroscience, Anaheim, CA., Nov. 6-10, 1977.) P.342.

Crowley, W.R., O'Donohue, T.L., and Jacobwitz, D.M. (1978): Changes in catecholamine content in discrete brain nuclei during the estrous cycle of the rat. *Brain Res.* 147-326.

Czaja, J.A. and Goy, R.W. (1975): Ovarian hormones and food intake in female guinea pigs and rhesus monkeys. *Horm. Behav.* 6:329-349.

Dantchakoff, V. (1941): *Der Aufbau des Geschlechts beim hoeheren Wirbeltier.* Jena: Gustav Fischer.

Darrah, H.K., MacKinnon, P.C.B., and Rogers, A.W. (1961): Sexual differentiation in the brain of the neonatal rat. *J. Physiol.* 218: 22P-23P.

Dattwyler, R.J., Murgita, R.A., and Tomasi, T.B., Jr. (1975): Binding of alpha-foetoprotein to murine cells. *Nature* 256:656-657.

Davidson, J.M. (1969): Effects of estrogen on the sexual behavior of male rats. *Endocrinology* 84:1365-1372.

Davidson, J.M. and Bloch, G.J. (1969): Neuroendocrine aspects of male reproduction. *Biol. Reprod.* 1(Suppl. 1):67-92.

Davidson, J.M. and Levine, S. (1969): Progesterone and heterotypical sexual behavior in male rats. *J. Endocrinol.* 44:129-130.

Davies, I.J., Naftolin, F., Ryan, K.J., Fischman, J., and Siu, J. (1975): The affinity of catechol-estrogens for estrogen receptors in the pituitary and anterior hypothalamus of the rat. *Endocrinology* 97:554-557.

Davis, H., Porter, J.W., Burton, J., and Levine, S. (1976): Sex and strain differences in lever-press shock escape behavior. *Physiol. Psychol.* 4:351-356.

Davis, P.G. and Barfield, R.J. (1979): Activation of masculine sexual behavior by intracranial estradiol benzoate implants in male rats. *Neuroendocrinology* 28:217-227.

Dawood, M.Y. and Saxena, B.B. (1977): Testosterone and dihydrotestosterone in maternal and cord blood in amniotic fluid. *Am. J. Obstet. Gynecol.* 129:37-42.

DeBold, J.F. and Whalen, R.E. (1975): Differential sensitivity of mounting and lordosis control systems to early androgen treatment in male and female hamsters. *Horm. Behav.* 6:197-209.

Denef, C. and de Moor, P. (1972): Sexual differentiation of steroid metabolizing enzymes in the rat liver. Further studies on predetermination by testosterone at birth. *Endocrinology* 91:374-384.

Denef, C., Magnus, C., and McEwen, B. (1973): Sex differences and hormonal control of testosterone metabolism in rat pituitary and brain. *J. Endocrinol.* 59:605-621.

Dennis, M. (1972): Sex-dependent and sex-independent neural control of reactivity to electric footshock in the rat. *Exp. Neurol.* 37:256-268.

Dennis, M. (1976): VMH lesions and reactivity to electric shock in the rat: The effect of early testosterone level. *Physiol. Behav.* 17:645-649.

Denti, A. and Epstein, E. (1972): Sex differences in the acquisition of two kinds of avoidance behavior in rats. *Physiol. Behav.* 8:611-615.

Diamond, M. (1966): Progesterone inhibition of normal sexual behavior in the male guinea pig. *Nature* 209:1322-1324.

Dilger, W.C. (1962): The behavior of lovebirds. *Sci. Am.* 206:88-98.

Döcke, F. and Dörner, G. (1975): Anovulation in adult female rats after neonatal intracerebral implantation of oestrogen. *Endokrinologie* 65:375-377.

Doerr, P., Pirke, K.M., Kockott, G., and Dittmar, F. (1976): Further studies on sex hormones in male homosexuals. *Arch. Gen. Psychiatry* 33:611-614.

Dohler, K.D. and Wuttke, W. (1975): Changes in levels of serum gonadotropins, prolactin, and gonadal steroids in prepubertal male and female rats. *Endocrinology* 97:898-907.

Domm, L.V. (1939): Modifications in sex and secondary sexual characters in birds. *In: Sex and Internal Secretions.* 2nd Ed. Allen, E., Danforth, C.H., and Doisy, E.A., eds. Baltimore: Williams and Wilkins, pp. 227-327.

Dörner, G. (1972): *Sexualhormonabhängige Gehirndifferenzierung und Sexualität.* New York: Springer-Verlag.

Dörner, G. (1974): Environment-dependent brain differentiation and fundamental processes of life. *Acta Biol. Med. Ger.* 33:129-148.

Dörner, G. (1975): Problems and terminology of functional teratology. *Acta Biol. Med. Ger.* 34:1093-1095.

Dörner, G. (1976): *Hormones and Brain Differentiation.* Amsterdam: Elsevier/North-Holland Biomedical Press.

Dörner, G. (1977): Hormone dependent differentiation, maturation and function of the brain and sexual behavior. *Endokrinologie* 69:306-320.

Dörner, G., Döcke, F., and Hinz, G. (1971): Paradoxical effects of estrogen on brain differentiation. *Neuroendocrinology* 7:146-155.

Dörner, G., Döcke, F., and Moustafa, S. (1968): Differential localization of a male and a female hypothalamic mating centre. *J. Reprod. Fertil.* 17:583-586.

Dörner, G. and Fatschel, J. (1970): Wirkungen neonatal verabreichter Androgene und Antiandrogene auf Sexualverhalten und Fertilität von Rattenweibchen. *Endokrinologie* 56: 29-48.

Dörner, G., Hect, K., and Hinz, G. (1976): Teratopsychogenetic effects apparently produced by nonphysiological neurotransmitter concentrations during brain differentiation. *Endokrinologie* 68:1-5.

Dörner, G. and Hinz, G. (1975): Androgen dependent brain differentiation and life span. *Endokrinologie* 65:378-380.

Dörner, G. and Hinz, G. (1978): Apparent effects of neurotransmitters on sexual differentiation of the brain without mediation of sex hormones. *Endokrinologie* 71:104-108.

Dörner, G., Hinz, G., Döcke, F., and Tönjes, R. (1977a): Effects of psychotrophic drugs on brain differentiation in female rats. *Endokrinologie* 70:113-123.

Dörner, G., Rohde, W., and Schnorr, D. (1975a): Evocability of a slight positive oestrogen feedback action on LH secretion in castrated and oestrogen-primed men. *Endokrinologie* 66:373-376.

Dörner, G., Rohde, W., Stahl, F., Krell, L., and Masius, W.G. (1975b): A neuroendocrine predisposition for homosexuality in men. *Arch. Sex. Behav.* 4:1-8.

Dörner, G., Stahl, F., Rohde, W., Göretzlehner, G., Witkowski, R., and Saffert, H. (1977b): Sex-specific testosterone and FSH concentrations in amniotic fluids of mid-pregnancy. *Endokrinologie* 70:86-88.

Dörner, G. and Staudt, J. (1968): Structural changes in the preoptic anterior hypothalamic area of the male rat, following neonatal castration and androgen substitution. *Neuroendocrinology* 3:136-140.

Dörner, G. and Staudt, J. (1969a): Perinatal structural sex differentiation of the hypothalamus in rats. *Neuroendocrinology* 5:103-106.

Dörner, G. and Staudt, J. (1969b): Structural changes in the hypothalamic ventromedial nucleus of the male rat following neonatal castration and androgen treatment. *Neuroendocrinology* 4:278-281.

Dörner, G., Staudt, J., Wenzel, J., Kvetňanský, R., and Murgaš, K. (1977c): Further evidence of teratogenic effects apparently produced by neurotransmitters during brain differentiation. *Endokrinologie* 70:326-330.

Doughty, C., Booth, J.E., McDonald, P.G., and Parrott, R.F. (1975a): Effects of oestradiol-17β, oestradiol benzoate and the synthetic oestrogen RU2858 on sexual differentiation in the neonatal female rat. *J. Endocrinol.* 67:419-424.

Doughty, C., Booth, J.E., McDonald, P.G., and Parrott, R.F. (1975b): Inhibition, by the anti-oestrogen MER-25, of defeminization induced by the synthetic oestrogen RU2858. *J. Endocrinol.* 67:459-460.

Doughty, C. and McDonald, P.G. (1974): Hormonal control of sexual differentiation of the hypothalamus in the neonatal female rat. *Differentiation* 2:275-285.

Dubuc, P. (1976): Body weight regulation in female rats following neonatal testosterone. *Acta Endocrinol.* 81:215-224.

Duck-Chong, C.J., Pollak, K., and North, R.J. (1964): The relation between the intracellular ribonucleic acid distribution and amino acid incorporation in the liver of the developing chick embryo. *J. Cell Biol.* 20:25-35.

Dunlap, J.L., Gerall, A.A., and Carlton, S.F. (1978): Evaluation of prenatal androgen and ovarian secretions on receptivity in female and male rats. *J. Comp. Physiol. Psychol.* 92: 280-288.

Dunlap, J.L., Gerall, A.A., and Hendricks, S.E. (1972): Female receptivity in neonatally castrated males as a function of age and experience. *Physiol. Behav.* 8:21-23.

Dunlap, J.L., Gerall, A.A., and McLean, L.D. (1973): Enhancement of female receptivity in neonatally castrated males by prepuberal ovarian transplants. *Physiol. Behav.* 10:701-705.

Dunlap, J.L., Preis, L.K., and Gerall, A.A. (1972): Compensatory ovarian hypertrophy as a function of age and neonatal androgenization. *Endocrinology.* 90:1309-1314.

Dyer, R.G., MacLeod, N.K., and Ellendorff, F. (1976): Electrophysiological evidence for sexual dimorphism and synaptic convergence in the preoptic anterior hypothalamic areas of the rat. *Proc. Roy. Soc. B* 193:421-440.

Dzwillo, M. von (1962): Uber kunstiliche Erzengung funtioneller Mannchen weiblichen Genotyps bei *Lebistes reticulatus. Biol. Zentralbl.* 81:575-584.

Eaton, G.G. (1976): The social order of Japanese macaques. *Sci. Am.* 235 (4):96-106.

Edwards, D.A. (1968): Mice: Fighting by neonatally androgenized females. *Science* 161: 1027-1028.

Edwards, D.A. (1969): Early androgen stimulation and aggressive behavior in male and female mice. *Physiol. Behav.* 4:333-338.

Edwards, D.A. (1970): Post-neonatal androgenization and adult aggressive behavior in female mice. *Physiol. Behav.* 5:465-467.

Edwards, D.A. (1971): Neonatal administration of androstenedione, testosterone or testosterone propionate: Effects on ovulation, sexual receptivity, and aggressive behavior in female mice. *Physiol. Behav.* 6:223-228.

Edwards, D.A. and Burge, K.G. (1971): Early androgen treatment and male and female sexual behavior in mice. *Horm. Behav.* 2:49-58.

Edwards, D.A. and Thompson, M.L. (1970): Neonatal androgenization and estrogenization and the hormonal induction of sexual receptivity in rats. *Physiol. Behav.* 5:115-119.

Eguchi, Y., Sakamoto, Y., Arishima, K., Morikawa, Y., and Hashimoto, Y. (1975): Hypothalamic control of the pituitary-testicular relation in fetal rats: measurement of collective volume of Leydig cells. *Endocrinology* 96:504-507.

Ehrhardt, A.A. (1973): Maternalism in fetal hormonal and related syndromes. *In: Contemporary Sexual Behavior: Critical Issues in the 1970's.* Zubin, J. and Money, J., eds. Baltimore: Johns Hopkins University Press, pp. 99-115.

Ehrhardt, A.A. (1974): Androgens in prenatal development: behavior changes in non-human primates and men. *In: Advances in the Biosciences, Vol. 13. Hormones and Embryonic Development.* Raspe, G., ed. New York: Pergamon Press, pp. 153-162.

Ehrhardt, A.A. (1975): Prenatal hormonal exposure and psychosexual differentiation. *In: Topics in Psychoendocrinology.* Sachar, E.J., ed. New York: Grune and Stratton, pp. 67-82.

Ehrhardt, A.A. (1975): Psychological correlates of abnormal pubertal development. *J. Clin. Endocrinol. Metab.* 4:207-222.

Ehrhardt, A.A. (1977a): Behavioral sequelae of prenatal hormone exposure in animals and man. Paper presented at American College of Neuropharmacology Symposium, New Orleans, Dec. 17, 1976.

Ehrhardt, A.A. (1977b): Prenatal androgenization and human psychosexual behavior. *In: Handbook of Sexology.* Money, J. and Musaph, H., eds. Amsterdam: Excerpta Medica, pp. 245-257.

Ehrhardt, A.A. and Baker, S.W. (1974): Fetal androgens, human CNS differentiation, and behavior sex differences. *In: Sex Differences in Behavior.* Friedman, R.C., Richart, R.M., and Vande Wiele, R.L., eds. New York: John Wiley and Sons, Inc., pp. 53-76.

Ehrhardt, A.A., Greenberg, N., and Money, J. (1970): Female gender identity and absence of fetal gonadal hormones: Turner's syndrome. *Johns Hopkins Med. J.* 126:237-248.

Ehrhardt, A.A., Grisanti, G.C., and Meyer-Bahlburg, H.F.L. (1977): Prenatal exposure to medroxyprogesterone acetate (MPA) in girls. *Psychoneuroendocrinology* 2:391-398.

Ehrhardt, A.A. and Money, J. (1967): Progestin-induced hermaphroditism: IQ and psychosexual identity in a study of ten girls. *J. Sex Res.* 3:83-100.

Eisenberg, L. (1972): The *human* nature of human nature. *Science* 176:123-128.

Eleftheriou, B.E., Bailey, D.W., and Denenberg, V.H. (1974): Genetic analysis of fighting behavior in mice. *Physiol. Behav.* 13:773-777.

Emery, D.E. and Sachs, B.D. (1975): Ejaculatory pattern in female rats without androgen treatment. *Science* 190:484-485.

Epple, G. (1972): Social behavior of laboratory groups of *Saguinus fuscicollis. In: Saving the Lion Marmoset.* Bridgewater, D.D., ed. Wheeling, W.Va.: The Wild Animal Propagation Trust, pp. 50-58.

Erpino, M.J. and Chappelle, T.C. (1973): Interactions between androgens and progesterone in mediation of aggression in the mouse. *Horm. Behav.* 2:265-272.

Eskay, R.L., Oliver, C., Grollman, D., and Porter, J.C. (1974): Immunoreactive LH-RH and TRH in the fetal, neonatal and adult rat brain. *In: Program and Abstracts of the Endocrinological Society, 56th Annual Meeting, Atlanta, GA,* P. H83. (Abstr.)

Farrell, A., Gerall, A.A., and Alexander, M.J. (1977): Age-related decline in receptivity in normal, neonatally androgenized female and male hamsters. *Exp. Aging Res.* 3:117-128.

Feder, H.H. (1967): Specificity of testosterone and estradiol in the differentiating neonatal rat. *Anat. Rec.* 157:79-86.

Feder, H.H., Naftolin, F., and Ryan, K.J. (1974): Male and female sexual responses in male rats given estradiol benzoate and 5α-androstan-17β-ol-3-one propionate. *Endocrinology* 94:136-141.

Fein, R. (1974): Men's experiences before and after the birth of the first child: Dependence, marital sharing and anxiety. Doctoral Dissertation, Harvard University, Cambridge, MA.

Feldman, S.C. and Bloch, E. (1977): Developmental pattern of testosterone synthesis by fetal rat testis in response to LH. *Endocrinology* 102:999-1007.

Fels, E. and Bosch, L.R. (1971): Effect of prenatal administration of testosterone on ovarian function in rats. *Am. J. Obstet. Gynecol.* 111:964-969.

Ferin, M., Zimmering, P.E., Lieberman, S., and Vande Wiele, R.L. (1968): Inactivation of the biological effects of exogenous and endogenous estrogens by antibodies to 17β-estradiol. *Endocrinology* 83:565-571.

Field, P.M. and Sherlock, D.A. (1975): Golgi studies of the sexually differentiated part of the preoptic area in the rat. *In: Golgi Centennial Symposium: Perspectives in Neurobiology.* Santini, M., ed. New York: Raven Press, pp. 143-146.

Fishman, J. and Norton, B. (1975): Catechol estrogen formation in the central nervous system of the rat. *Endocrinology* 96:1054-1058.

Flerko, B. and Mess, B. (1968): Reduced oestradiol-binding capacity of androgen sterilized rats. *Acta Physiol. Acad. Sci. Hung.* 33:111-113.

Flerko, B., Mess, B., and Illei-Donohoffer, A. (1969): On the mechanism of androgen sterilization. *Neuroendocrinology* 4:164-169.

Floody, O.R. and Pfaff, D.W. (1977): Aggressive behavior in female hamsters: The hormonal basis for fluctuations in female aggressiveness correlated with estrous state. *J. Comp. Physiol. Psychol.* 91:443-464.

Foote, C.L. (1964): Intersexuality in amphibians. *In: Intersexuality in Vertebrates Including Man.* Armstrong, C.N. and Marshall, A.J., eds. London: Academic Press, pp. 273-284.

Fox, T.O. (1975a): Androgen- and estrogen-binding macromolecules in developing mouse brain: Biochemical and genetic evidence. *Proc. Nat. Acad. Sci.* 72:4303-4307.

Fox, T.O. (1975b): Oestradiol receptor of neonatal mouse brain. *Nature* 258:441-444.

Fox, T.O. (1977a): Conversion of the hypothalamic estradiol receptor to the nuclear form. *Brain Res.* 120:580-583.

Fox, T.O. (1977b): Estradiol and testosterone binding in normal and mutant mouse cerebellum: biochemical and cellular specificity. *Brain Res.* 128:263-273.

Fox, T.O. and Johnston, C. (1974): Estradiol receptors from mouse brain and uterus: binding to DNA. *Brain Res.* 77:330-336.

Fox, T.O., Vito, C.C., and Wieland, S.J. (1978): Estrogen and androgen receptor proteins in embryonic and neonatal brain: hypotheses for roles in sexual differentiation and behavior. *Am. Zool.* 18:525-537.

Fricke, H. and Fricke, S. (1977): Monogamy and sex change by aggressive dominance in coral reef fish. *Nature* 266:830-832.

Friedmann, H., Kiff, L.F., and Rothstein, S.I. (1977): A further contribution to knowledge of the host relations of the parasitic cowbirds. *Smithson. Contrib. Zool.* 235:1-75.

Frith, H.J. (1964): Megapode. *In: A New Dictionary of Birds.* Landsborough, T.A., ed. London: Nelson, pp. 451-453.

Gallien, L.G. (1965): Genetic control of sexual differentiation in vertebrates. *In: Organogenesis.* Dehaan, R.L. and Ursprung, H., eds. New York: Holt, Rinehart and Winston, pp. 583-610.

Gallien, L.G. (1967): Developments in sexual organogenesis. *In: Advances in Morphogenesis, Vol. 6.* Abercrombie, M. and Brachet, J., eds. New York: Academic Press, pp. 259-317.

Gandelman, R. vom Saal, F.S., and Reinisch, J.M. (1977): Contiguity to male foetuses affects morphology and behaviour of female mice. *Nature* 266:722-724.

Gartlan, J.S. (1968): Structure and function in primate society. *Folia Primatologica* 8:89-120.

Gay, V.L. (1975): Ineffectiveness of DHT treatment in producing increased serum DHT in orchidectomized rats: evidence for rapid *in vivo* metabolism of DHT to androstanediol. *Fed. Proc.* 34:303. (Abstr.)

Gehring, U., Tomkins, G.M., and Ohno, S. (1971): Effect of the androgen-insensitivity mutation on a cytoplasmic receptor for dihydrotestosterone. *Nature New Biol.* 232:106-107.

Gentry, R.T. and Wade, G.N. (1976a): Androgenic control of food intake and body weight in male rats. *J. Comp. Physiol. Psychol.* 90:18-25.

Gentry, R.T. and Wade, G.N. (1976b): Sex differences in sensitivity of food intake, body weight and running-wheel activity to ovarian steroids in rats. *J. Comp. Physiol. Psychol.* 90:747-754.

George, F.W., Tobleman, W.T., Milewich, L., and Wilson, J.D. (1978): Aromatase activity in the developing rabbit brain. *Endocrinology* 102:86-91.

Gerall, A.A. (1966): Hormonal factors influencing masculine behavior of female guinea pigs. *J. Comp. Physiol. Psychol.* 62:365-369.

Gerall, A.A. (1967): Effects of early postnatal androgen and estrogen injections of the estrous activity cycles and mating behavior of rats. *Anat. Rec.* 157:97-104.

Gerall, A.A. and Dunlap, J.L. (1971): Evidence that the ovaries of the neonatal rat secrete active substances. *J. Endocrinol.* 50:529-530.

Gerall, A.A. and Dunlap, J.L. (1973): The effect of experience and hormones on the initial receptivity in female and male rats. *Physiol. Behav.* 10:851-854.

Gerall, A.A. and Dunlap, J.L. (1973): Time dependent changes induced by neonatal androgen. *In: Corticothalamic Projections and Sensorimotor Activities.* (BIS Conference Report Number 16.) Los Angeles: University of California Brain Information Service, pp. 38-41.

Gerall, A.A., Dunlap, J.L., and Hendricks, S.E. (1972a): Effect of ovarian secretions on female behavioral potentiality in the rat. *J. Comp. Physiol. Psychol.* 82:449-465.

Gerall, A.A., Dunlap, J.L., and Wagner, R.A. (1976): Effects of dihydrotestosterone and gonadotropins on the development of female behavior. *Physiol. Behav.* 17:121-126.

Gerall, A.A., Dunlap, J.L., Sonntag, W.E. (1979): Reproduction in aging normal and neonatally androgenized female rats. *J. Comp. Physiol. Psychol.* (In press)

Gerall, A.A., Hendricks, S.E., Johnson, L.L., and Bounds, T.W. (1967): Effects of early castration in male rats on adult sexual behavior. *J. Comp. Physiol. Psychol.* 64:206-212.

Gerall, A.A. and Kenney, A.McM. (1970): Neonatally androgenized females' responsiveness to estrogen and progesterone. *Endocrinology.* 87:560-566.

Gerall, A.A., McMurray, M.M., and Farrell, A. (1975): Suppression of the development of female hamster behaviour by implants of testosterone and non-aromatizable androgens administered neonatally. *J. Endocrinol.* 67:439-445.

Gerall, A.A., Stone, L.S., and Hitt, J.C. (1972b): Neonatal androgen depresses female responsiveness to estrogen. *Physiol. Behav.* 8:17-20.

Gerall, A.A. and Thiel, A.R. (1975): Effects of perinatal gonadal secretions on parameters of receptivity and weight gain in hamsters. *J. Comp. Physiol. Psychol.* 89:580-589.

Gerall, A.A. and Ward, L.L. (1966): Effects of prenatal exogenous androgen on the sexual behavior of the female albino rat. *J. Comp. Physiol. Psychol.* 62:370-375.

Gethmann, U. and Knuppen, R. (1976): Effect of 2-hydroxyestrone on lutropin (LH) and follitropin (FSH) secretion in the ovariectomized primed rat. *Hoppe-Seyler's Z. Physiol. Chem.* 357:1011-1013.

Gil, D.G. (1970): Physical abuse of children. *Pediatrics* 45: 510-511.

Gil, D.G. (1970): *Violence Against Children: Physical Child Abuse in the United States.* Cambridge, MA: Harvard University Press.

Giles, H.R., Lox, C.D., Heine, M.W., and Christian, C.D. (1974): Intrauterine fetal sex determination by radioimmunoassay of amniotic fluid testosterone. *Gynecol. Invest.* 5:317-323.

Gilliard, E.T. (1969): *Birds of Paradise and Bower Birds.* New York: Natural History Press.

Gladue, B.A. and Clemens, L.G. (1978): Androgenic influences on feminine sexual behavior in male and female rats: defeminization blocked by prenatal antiandrogen treatment. *Endocrinology* 103:1702-1709.

Globus, A. Rosenzweig, M.R., Bennett, E.L., and Diamond, M.C. (1973): Effects of differential experience on dendritic spine counts in rat cerebral cortex. *J. Comp. Fhysiol. Psychol.* 82:175-181.

Globus, A. and Scheibel, A.B. (1967): The effect of visual deprivation on cortical neurons: a Golgi study. *Exp. Neurol.* 19:331-345.

Goldfoot, D.A., Feder, H.H., and Goy, R.W. (1969): Development of bisexuality in the male rat treated neonatally with androstenedione. *J. Comp. Physiol. Psychol.* 67:41-45.

Goldfoot, D.A. and van der Werff ten Bosch, J.J. (1975): Mounting behavior of female guinea pigs after prenatal and adult administration of the propionates of testosterone, dihydrotestosterone, and androstanediol. *Horm. Behav.* 6:139-148.

Goldfoot, D.A. and Wallen, K. (1978): Development of gender role behaviors in heterosexual and isosexual groups of infant rhesus monkeys. *In: Recent Advances in Primatology, Vol. 1. Behaviour.* New York: Academic Press, pp. 155-159.

Goldman, P.S., Crawford, H.T., Stokes, L.P., Galkin, T.W., and Rosvold, H.E. (1974): Sex-dependent behavioral effects of cerebral cortical lesions in the developing rhesus monkey. *Science* 186:540-542.

Goldstein, J.L. and Wilson, J.D. (1972): Studies on the pathogenesis of pseudohermaphroditism in the mouse with testicular feminization. *J. Clin. Invest.* 51:1647-1658.

Goldstein, J.L. and Wilson, J.D. (1975): Genetic and hormonal control of male sexual differentiation. *J. Cell Physiol.* 85:365-378.

Gorski, R.A. (1966): Localization and sexual differentiation of the nervous structures which regulate ovulation. *J. Reprod. Fertil. Suppl.* 1:67-88.

Gorski, R.A. (1967): Localization of the neural control of luteinization in the feminine male rat (FALE). *Anat. Rec.* 157:63-69.

Gorski, R.A. (1971): Gonadal hormones and the perinatal development of neuroendocrine function. *In: Frontiers in Neuroendocrinology.* Martini, L. and Ganong, W.F., eds. New York: Oxford University Press, pp. 237-290.

Gorski, R.A. (1973): Perinatal effects of sex steroids on brain development and function. *Prog. Brain Res.* 39:149-162.

Gorski, R.A. (1974a): Barbiturates and sexual differentiation of the brain. *In: Narcotics and the Hypothalamus.* Zimmerman, E. and George, R., eds. New York: Raven Press, pp. 197-211.

Gorski, R.A. (1974b): The neuroendocrine regulation of sexual behavior. *In: Advances in Psychobiology, Vol. II.* Newton, G. and Riesen, A.H., eds. New York: John Wiley and Sons, pp. 1-58.

Gorski, R.A., Gordon, J.H., Shryne, J.E., and Southam, A.M. (1978): Evidence for a morphological sex difference within the medial preoptic area of the rat brain. *Brain Res.* 148: 333-346.

Gorski, R.A., Harlan, R.E., and Christensen, L.W. (1977): Perinatal hormonal exposure and the development of neuroendocrine processes. *J. Toxicol. Environ. Health* 3:97-121.

Gorski, R.A. and Shryne, J. (1972): Intracerebral antibiotics and androgenization of the neonatal female rat. *Neuroendocrinology* 10:109-120.

Gorski, R.A. and Wagner, J.W. (1965): Gonadal activity and sexual differentiation of the hypothalamus. *Endocrinology* 76:226-239.

Gottlieb, D.I. and Cowan, W.M. (1972): Evidence for a temporal factor in the occupation of available synaptic sites during development of the dentate gyrus. *Brain Res.* 41:452-456.

Gottlieb, H., Gerall, A.A., and Thiel, A.R. (1974): Receptivity in female hamsters following neonatal testosterone, testosterone propionate, and MER-25. *Physiol. Behav.* 12:61-68.

Goy, R.W. (1966): Role of androgens in the establishment and regulation of behavioral sex differences in mammals. *J. Anim. Sci. Suppl.* 25:21-35.

Goy, R.W. (1968): Organizing effects of androgen on the behaviour of rhesus monkeys. *In: Endocrinology and Human Behaviour.* Michael, R.P., ed. London: Oxford University Press, pp. 12-31.

Goy, R.W. (1970a): Early hormonal influences on the development of sexual and sex-related behavior. *In: The Neurosciences: Second Study Program.* Schmitt, F.O., Editor-in-chief. New York: Rockefeller University Press, pp. 196-206.

Goy, R.W. (1970b): Experimental control of psychosexuality. *Phil. Trans. R. Soc. B* 259:149-162.

Goy, R.W. (1978): Development of play and mounting behaviour in female rhesus virilized prenatally with esters of testosterone and dihydrotestosterone. *In: Recent Advances in Primatology, Vol. 1. Behaviour.* Chivers, D.J. and Herbert, J., eds. London: Academic Press, pp. 449-462.

Goy, R.W., Bridson, W.E., and Young, W.C. (1964): Period of maximal susceptibility of the prenatal female guinea pig to masculinizing actions of testosterone propionate. *J. Comp. Physiol. Psychol.* 57:166-174.

Goy, R.W. and Goldfoot, D.A. (1973): Hormonal influences on sexually dimorphic behavior. *In: Handbook of Physiology, Endocrinology II, Part 1.* Greep, R.O. and Astwood, E.B., eds. Baltimore: Williams and Wilkins, pp. 169-186.

Goy, R.W. and Goldfoot, D.A. (1974): Experimental and hormonal factors influencing development of sexual behavior in the male rhesus monkey. *In: The Neurosciences: Third Study Program.* Schmitt, F.O. and Worden, F.G., Editors-in-chief. Cambridge, Mass.: M.I.T. Press, pp. 571-581.

Goy, R.W. and Goldfoot, D.A. (1975): Neuroendocrinology: animal models and problems of human sexuality. *Arch. Sex. Behav.* 4:405-420.

Goy, R.W. and Jakway, J.S. (1959): The inheritance of patterns of sexual behaviour in female guinea pigs. *Anim. Behav.* 7:142-149.

Goy, R.W. and Phoenix, C.H. (1971): The effects of testosterone propionate administered before birth on the development of behavior in genetic female rhesus monkeys. *In: Steroid Hormones and Brain Function.* Sawyer, C. and Gorski, R., eds. Berkeley: University of California Press, pp. 193-201.

Goy, R.W. and Resko, J.A. (1972): Gonadal hormones and behavior of normal and pseudohermaphroditic nonhuman female primates. *Rec. Prog. Horm. Res.* 28:707-733.

Goy, R.W. and Wallen, K. (1979): Experimental variables influencing play, footclasp mounting, and adult sexual competence in male rhesus monkeys. *Psychoneuroendocrinology* 4:1-12.

Goy, R.W., Wolf, J.E., and Eisele, S.G. (1977): Experimental female hermaphroditism in rhesus monkeys: anatomical and psychological characteristics. *In: Handbook of Sexology.* Money, J. and Musaph, H., eds. Amsterdam: Excerpta Medica, pp. 139-156.

Goy, R.W. and Young, W.C. (1957): Strain differences in the behavioral responses of female guinea pigs to alpha-estradiol benzoate and progesterone. *Behaviour* 10:340-354.

Grady, K.L., Phoenix, C.H., and Young, W.C. (1965): Role of the developing rat testis in differentiation of the neural tissues mediating mating behavior. *J. Comp. Physiol. Psychol.* 59:176-182.

Grasso, J.A., Swift, H., and Ackerman, G.A. (1962): Observation on the development of erythrocytes in mammalian fetal liver. *J. Cell Biol.* 14:235-254.

Grave, G.D. (1977): *Thyroid Hormones and Brain Development.* New York: Raven Press.

Gray, G.D., Davis, H.N., and Dewsbury, D.A. (1976): Masculine sexual behavior in male and female rats following perinatal manipulation of androgen: effects of genital anesthetization and sexual experience. *Horm. Behav.* 7:317-329.

Gray, J.A. (1971): Sex differences in emotional behaviour in mammals including man: Endocrine bases. *Acta Psychol.* 35:29-46.

Gray, J.A., Levine, S., and Broadhurst, P.L. (1965): Gonadal hormone injections in infancy and adult emotional behavior. *Anim. Behav.* 13:33-45.

Gray, P. (1977): Effect of the estrous cycle on conditioned avoidance in mice. *Horm. Behav.* 8:235-241.

Greenough, W.T. (1975): Experimental modification of the developing brain. *Am. Sci.* 63: 37-46.

Greenough, W.T., Carter, C.S., Ackerman, T., Reeder, R., Mateer, J., Reeder, T., Lyerla, E., Bohnsak, M., McCabe, P., Suits, C., and DeVoogd, T.J. (1977a): Sexual dimorphism in dendritic pattern in basal forebrain regions of intact adult hamsters. *In: Neuroscience Abstracts, Vol. III.* (Seventh Annual Meeting of the Society for Neuroscience, Anaheim, CA, Nov. 6-10, 1977.) P. 345

Greenough, W.T., Carter, C.S., Steerman, C., and DeVoogd, T.J. (1977b): Sex differences in dendritic patterns in hamster preoptic area. *Brain Res.* 126:63-72.

Greenough, W.T., Volkmar, F.R., and Juraska, J.M. (1973): Effects of rearing complexity on dendritic branching in frontolateral and temporal cortex of the rat. *Exp. Neurol.* 41: 371-378.

Gregory, E. (1975): Comparison of postnatal CNS development between male and female rats. *Brain Res.* 99:152-156.

Griffin, J.E., Punyashtihti, K., and Wilson, J.D. (1976): Dihydrotestosterone binding by cultured human fibroblasts. Comparison of cells from control subjects and from patients with hereditary male pseudohermaphroditism due to androgen resistance. *J. Clin. Invest.* 57: 1342-1351.

Gutstein, J. (1978): Behavioural correlates of male dispersal in patas monkeys. *In: Recent Advances in Primatology, Vol 1, Behaviour.* Chiver, D.J. and Herbert, J., eds. London: Academic Press, pp. 79-82.

Hackmann, E. and Reinboth, R. (1974): Delimitation of the critical stage of hormone-influenced sex differentiation in *Hemihaplochromis multicolor.* (Hilgendorf) (Cichlidae). *Gen. Comp. Endocrinol.* 22:42-53.

Haffen, K. (1975): Sex differentiation of avian gonads in vitro. *Am. Zool.* 15:257-272.

Hamburg, D.A. (1974): Coping behavior in life-threatening circumstances. *Psychother. Psychosom.* 23:13-25.

Hamburg, D.A. (1974): The psychobiology of sex differences: An evolutionary perspective. *In: Sex Differences in Behavior.* Friedman, R.C., Richart, R.M., and Vande Wiele, R.L., eds. New York: John Wiley and Sons, Inc., pp. 373-392.

Harlan, R.E. and Gorski, R.A. (1977): Correlations between ovarian sensitivity, vaginal cyclicity and luteinizing hormone and prolactin secretion in lightly androgenized rats. *Endocrinology* 101:750-759.

Harlan, R.E. and Gorski, R.A. (1978): Effects of postpubertal ovarian steroids on reproductive function and sexual differentiation of lightly androgenized rats. *Endocrinology* 102:1716-1724.

Harrell, L.E. and Balagura, S. (1975): Influence of ovarian hormones on the recovery period following lateral hypothalamic lesions. *J. Comp. Physiol. Psychol.* 88:194-201.

Harris, G.W. (1964): Sex hormones, brain development and brain function. *Endocrinology* 75:627-648.

Harris, G.W. and Jacobson, D. (1952): Functional grafts of the anterior pituitary gland. *Proc. R. Soc. B* 139:263-276.

Harris, G.W. and Levine, S. (1965): Sexual differentiation of the brain and its experimental control. *J. Physiol.* 181:379-400.

Hart, B.L. (1972): Manipulation of neonatal androgen: effects on sexual responses and penile development in male rats. *Physiol. Behav.* 8:841-845.

Hart, B.L. (1977): Neonatal dihydrotestosterone and estrogen stimulation: effects on sexual behavior of male rats. *Horm. Behav.* 8:193-200.

Hatton, G.I. (1976): Nucleus circularis: Is it an osmoreceptor in the brain? *Brain Res. Bull.* 1:123-131.

Hayashi, S. (1974): Failure of intrahypothalamic implants of antiestrogen, MER-25, to inhibit androgen-sterilization in female rats. *Endocrinol. Jpn.* 21:453-457.

Hayashi, S. (1976): Failure of intrahypothalamic implants of an estrogen antagonist, ethamoxytriphetol (MER-25), to block neonatal androgen-sterilization. *Proc. Soc. Exp. Biol. Med.* 152:389-392.

Hayashi, S. and Gorski, R.A. (1974): Critical exposure time for androgenization by intracranial crystals of testosterone propionate in neonatal female rats. *Endocrinology* 94:1161-1167.

Hays, H. (1972): Polyandry in the spotted sandpiper. *Living Bird* 11:43-58.

Hendricks, S.E. (1969): Influence of neonatally administered hormones and early gonadectomy on rats' sexual behavior. *J. Comp. Physiol. Psychol.* 69:408-413.

Hendricks, S.E. (1972): Androgen modification of behavioral responsiveness to estrogen in the male rat. *Horm. Behav.* 3:47-54.

Hendricks, S.E. and Duffy, J.A. (1974): Ovarian influences on the development of sexual behavior in neonatally androgenized rats. *Dev. Psychobiol.* 7:297-303.

Hendricks, S.E. and Gerall, A.A. (1970): Effect of neonatally administered estrogen on development of male and female rats. *Endocrinology* 87:435-439.

Hendricks, S.E. and Weltin, M. (1976): Effect of estrogen given during various periods of prepuberal life on the sexual behavior of rats. *Physiol. Psychol.* 4:105-110.

Henrik, E. and Gerall, A.A. (1976): Facilitation of receptivity in estrogen-primed rats during successive mating tests with progestins and methysergide. *J. Comp. Physiol. Psychol.* 90: 590-600.

Herbst, A.L., Kurman, R.J., Scully, R.E., and Poskanzen, D.C. (1972): Clear-cell adenocarcinoma of the genital tract in young females. *New Eng. J. Med.* 287:1259-1264.

Herrick, E.H. and Harris, J.O. (1957): Singing female canaries. *Science* 125:1299-1300.

Hinde, R.A. (1953): The conflict between drives in the courtship and copulation of the Chaffinch. *Behaviour* 5:1-31.

Hinde, R.A. (1965): Interaction of internal and external factors in integration of canary reproduction. *In: Sex and Behavior.* Beach, F.A., ed. New York: John Wiley and Sons, Inc., pp. 381-415.

Hinde, R.A. (1970): *Animal Behavior. A Synthesis of Ethology and Comparative Psychology.* New York: McGraw-Hill.

Hinde, R.A. and Steel, E. (1966): Integration of the reproductive behavior of female canaries. *Symp. Soc. Exp. Biol.* 20:401-426.

Hinman, F. (1951): Sexual trends in female pseudohermaphroditism. *J. Clin. Endocrinol. Metab.* 11:477-486.

Hirsch, S.M. and Bronstein, P.M. (1976): Ovariectomy fails to affect rats' quinine aversion. *Physiol. Behav.* 16:375-377.

Hitchcock, F.A. (1925): Studies in vigor. V. The comparative activity of male and female albino rats. *Am. J. Physiol.* 75:205-210.

Hjorth, I. (1970): Reproductive behavior in *Tetraonidae. Viltrevy* 7:184-596.

Hogan-Warburg, A.J. (1966): Social behavior of the ruff, *Philomachus pugnax* (L). *Ardea* 54:109-229.

Höhn, E.O. (1967): Observations on the breeding biology of Wilson's phalarope (*Steganopus tricolor*) in central Alberta. *Auk* 84:220-244.

Höhn, E.O. and Cheng, S.C. (1967): Gonadal hormones in Wilson's phalarope *Steganopus tricolor* and other birds in relation to plumage and sex behavior. *Gen. Comp. Endocrinol.* 8:1-11.

Holloway, R.L., Jr. (1966): Dendritic branching: some preliminary results of training and complexity in rat visual cortex. *Brain Res.* 2:393-396.

Holman, S.D. (1976): Neonatal androgen and mounting behavior in female house mice. *Anim. Behav.* 24:135-140.

Hooker, B.I. (1968): Birds. *In: Animal Communication.* Sebeok, T.A., ed. Bloomington, Ind.: Indiana University Press, pp. 311-337.

Howard, E. (1920): *Territory in Bird Life.* London: John Murray.

Hunt, G.L., Jr. and Hunt, M.W. (1977): Female-female pairing in Western gulls *Larus occidentalis* in Southern California. *Science* 196:1466-1467.

Hutchinson, R., Ulrich, R., and Azzin, N. (1965): Effects of age and related factors on the pain aggression reaction. *J. Comp. Physiol. Psychol.* 59:365-369.

Hutchison, J.B. (1967): Initiation of courtship by hypothalamic implants of testosterone propionate in castrated doves (*Sterptopelia risoria*). *Nature* 216:591-592.

Hutchison, J.B. (1975): Target cells for gonadal steroids in the brain: studies on steroid-sensitive mechanisms of behaviour. *In: Neural and Endocrine Aspects of Behaviour in Birds.* Wright, P., Caryl, P.G., and Vowles, D.M., eds., Amsterdam: Elsevier, pp. 123-137.

Huxley, J.S. (1914): The courtship-habits of the great crested grebe *Podiceps cristatus;* with an addition to the theory of sexual selection. *Proc. Zool. Soc.* 35:491-562. (Reprinted as *The Courtship of the Great Crested Grebe*, with a foreword by Desmond Morris, Cape Editions, London: Grossman.)

Ifft, J.D. (1972): An autoradiographic study of the time of final division of neurons in rat hypothalamic nuclei. *J. Comp. Neurol.* 144:193-204.

Ikard, W.L., Bennett, W.C., Lundin, R.W., and Trost, R.C. (1972): Acquisition and extinction of the conditioned avoidance response: a comparison between male rats and estrus and non-estrus female rats. *Psychol. Rec.* 22:249-254.

Imperato-McGinley, J., Guerrero, L., Gautier, T., and Peterson, R.E. (1974): Steroid 5α-reductase deficiency in man: an inherited form of male pseudohermaphroditism. *Science* 186:1213-1215.

Imperato-McGinley, J. and Peterson, R.E. (1976): Male pseudohermaphroditism: the complexities of male phenotypic development. *Am. J. Med.* 61:251-272.

Jenni, D.A. and Collier, G. (1972): Polyandry in the American jacana (*Jacana spinosa*). *Auk* 89:743-765.

Johnson, D.A. (1972): Developmental aspects of recovery following septal lesions in the infant rat. *J. Comp. Physiol. Psychol.* 78:311-348.

Joslyn, W.D. (1973): Androgen-induced social dominance in infant female rhesus monkeys. *J. Child Psychol. Psychiat.* 14:137-145.

Joslyn, W.D., Wallen, K., and Goy, R.W. (1976): Advancement of ovulation in the guinea-pig with exogenous progesterone and related effects on length of the oestrous cycle and life span of the corpus luteum. *J. Endocrinol.* 70:275-283.

Josso, N. (1972): Permeability of membranes to the müllerian-inhibiting substance synthesized by the human fetal testis *in vitro:* a clue to its biomedical nature. *J. Clin. Endocrinol.* 34:265-270.

Josso, N., Forest, M.G., and Picard, J.Y. (1975): Müllerian-inhibiting activity of calf fetal testes: relationship of testosterone and protein synthesis. *Biol. Reprod.* 13:163-167.

Jost, A. (1953): Problems of fetal endocrinology: The gonadal ahd hypophyseal hormones. *Rec. Prog. Horm. Res.* 8:379-418.

Jost, A. (1961): The role of fetal hormones in prenatal development. *Harvey Lec.* 55:201-226.

Jost, A. (1965): Gonadal hormones in sex differentiation of the mammalian fetus. *In: Organogenesis.* DeHahn, R.L. and Ursprung, H., eds. New York: Holt, Rinehart and Winston, Inc., pp. 611-628.

Jost, A. (1970): Hormonal factors in the sex differentiation of the mammalian foetus. *Phil. Trans. R. Soc. B* 259:119-130.

Jost, A. (1972): A new look at the mechanisms controlling sex differentiation in mammals. *Johns Hopkins Med. J.* 130:38-53.

Judd, H.L., Robinson, J.D., Young, P.E., and Jones, O.W. (1976): Amniotic fluid testosterone levels in mid-pregnancy. *Obstet. Gynecol.* 48:690-692.

Kanter, R.M., Jaffe, D., and Weisburg, D.K. (1975): Coupling, parenting and the presence of others: intimate relationships in communal households. *The Family Coordinator* 24: 433-452.

Kao, L.W.L., Perez-Lloret, A.P., and Weisz, J. (1977): Metabolism *in vitro* of dihydrostestosterone, 5α-androstane3alpha,17β-diol and its 3β-epimer, three metabolites of testosterone, by three of its target issues, the anterior pituitary, the medial basal hypothalamus and the seminiferous tubules. *J. Steroid Biochem.* 8:1109-1115.

Kao, L.W.L. and Weisz, J. (1975): Direct effect of testosterone and its 5α-reduced metabolites on pituitary LH and FSH release in vitro: change in pituitary responsiveness to hypothalamic extract. *Endocrinology* 96:253-260.

Karsch, F.J., Dierschke, D., and Knobil, E. (1973): Sexual differentiation of pituitary function: apparent difference between primates and rodents. *Science* 179:484-486.

Katzenellenbogen, B.S., Ferguson, E.R., and Lan, N.C. (1977): Fundamental differences in the action of estrogens and antiestrogens on the uterus: Comparison between compounds with similar duration of action. *Endocrinology* 100:1252-1259.

Kearly, R.C., van Hartesveldt, C., and Woodruff, M.L. (1974): Behavioral and hormonal effects of hippocampal lesions on male and female rats. *Physiol. Psychol.* 2:187-196.

Kemnitz, J.W., Goy, R.W., and Keesey, R.E. (1977): Effects of gonadectomy on hypothalamic obesity in male and female rats. *Int. J. Obesity* 1:259-270.

Kikuyama, S. (1966): Influence of thyroid hormone on the induction of persistent estrus by androgen in the rat. *Sci. Papers Coll. Gen. Ed.* 16:165-270.

Kikuyama, S. (1969): Alteration by neonatal hypothyroidism of the critical period for the induction of persistent estrus in the rat. *Endocrinol. Jpn.* 16:269-273.

Kim, C.K., Yen, S.S.C., and Bernirschke, K. (1972): Serum testosterone in fetal cattle. *Gen. Comp. Endocrinol.* 18:404-407.

Kincl, F.A. and Maqueo, M. (1965): Prevention by progesterone of steriod-induced sterility in neonatal male and female rats. *Endocrinology* 77:859-862.

Kincl, F.A., Pi, A.F., Maqueo, M., Lasso, L.H., Oriol, A., and Dorfman, R.I. (1965): Inhibition of sexual development in male and female rats treated with various steroids at the age of five days. *Acta Endocrinol.* 49:193-206.

King, J.C. and Gerall, A.A. (1976): Localization of luteinizing hormone-releasing hormone, *J. Histochem. Cytochem.* 24:829-845.

King, J.C., Parsons, J.A., Erlandsen, S.L., and Williams, T.H. (1974): Luteinizing hormone-releasing hormone (LH-RH) pathway of the rat hypothalamus revealed by the unlabeled antibody peroxidase-antiperoxidase method. *Cell Tiss. Res.* 153:211-217.

King, J.M. and Cox, V.C. (1973): The effects of estrogens on food intake and body weight following ventromedial hypothalamic lesions. *Physiol. Psychol.* 1:261-264.

Klaus, M.H., Jerauld, R., Kreger, N., et al. (1972): Maternal attachment. *New Eng. J. Med.* 286:460-463.

Klaus, M.H., Kennell, J.H., Plumb, N., and Zuehike, S. (1970): Human maternal behavior at first contact with her young. *Pediatrics* 46:187-192.

Kobayashi, F. and Gorski, R.A. (1970): Effects of antibiotics on androgenization of the neonatal female rat. *Endocrinology* 86:285-289.

Kobayashi, R.M. and Reed, K.C. (1977): Conversion of androgens to estrogens (aromatization) in discrete regions of the rat brain: Sexual differences and effects of castration. *In: Neuroscience Abstracts, Vol. III.* (Seventh Annual Meeting of the Society for Neuroscience, Anaheim, CA., Nov. 6-10, 1977.) P.348.

Kondo, C.Y. and Lorens, S.A. (1971): Sex differences in the effects of septal lesions. *Physiol. Behav.* 6:481-485.

Konishi, M. (1965): The role of auditory feedback in the control of vocalizations in the white-crowned sparrow. *Z. Tierpsychol.* 22:770-783.

Konishi, M. and Nottebohm, F. (1969): Experimental studies in the ontogeny of avian vocalizations. *In: Bird Vocalizations.* Hinde, R.A., ed. Cambridge: University of Cambridge Press, pp. 29-48.

Korenbrot, C.C., Paup, D.C., and Gorski, R.A. (1975): Effects of testosterone propionate or dihydrotestosterone propionate on plasma FSH and LH levels in neonatal rats and on sexual differentiation of the brain. *Endocrinology* 97:709-717.

Kornguth, S.E. and Scott, G. (1972): The role of climbing fibers in the formation of Purkinje cell dendrites. *J. Comp. Neurol.* 146:61-82.

Kozelka, A.W. and Gallagher, T.F. (1934): Effect of male hormone extracts, theelin and theelol, on the chick embryo. *Proc. Soc. Exp. Zool. Med.* 31:1143-1144.

Krasnoff, A. and Weston, L.M. (1976): Puberal status and sex differences: Activity and maze behavior in rats. *Dev. Psychobiol.* 9:261-269.

Krecek, J. (1973): Sex differences in salt taste: The effect of testosterone. *Physiol. Behav.* 10:683-688.

Krecek, J., Novakova, V., and Stibral, K. (1972): Sex differences in the taste preference for a salt solution in the rat. *Physiol. Behav.* 8:183-188.

Kulin, H.E. and Reiter, E.O. (1976): Gonadotropin and testosterone measurements after estrogen administration to adult men, prepubertal and pubertal boys, and men with hypogonadotropism: evidence for maturation of positive feedback in the male. *Pediatr. Res.* 10:46-51.

Kummer, H. (1971): *Primate Societies: Group Techniques of Ecological Adaptation.* Chicago: Aldine-Atherton, Inc.

Kunzig, H.J., Meyer, U., Schmitz-Roeckerath, B., and Broer, K.H. (1977): Influence of fetal sex on the concentration of amniotic fluid testosterone: Antenatal sex determination? *Arch. Gynaekol.* 223:75-84.

Lack, D. (1943): *The Life of the Robin.* London: Witherby.

Lade, B.I. and Thorpe, W.H. (1964): Dove songs as innately coded patterns of specific behaviour. *Nature* 202:366-368.

Ladosky, W. (1967): Anovulatory sterility in rats neonatally injected with stilbestrol. *Endokrilogie* 52:259-261.

Ladosky, W., Kesikowski, W.M., and Gaziri, I.F. (1970): Effect of a single injection of chlorpromazine into infant male rats on subsequent gonadotrophin secretion. *J. Endocrinol.* 48:151-156.

Lancaster, J.B. (1975): *Primate Behavior and the Emergence of Human Culture.* New York: Holt, Rinehart and Winston.

Landmesser, L. and Pilar, G. (1978): Interactions between neurons and their targets during in vivo synaptogenesis, *Fed. Proc.* 37:2016-2022.

Laron, Z. Pertzelan, A. Shurka, E., Galatzer, A., Gil, R., and Frisch, M. (1974): Physiological and psychological aspects at puberty of patients with congenital adrenocortical virilism (CAV). *In: Endocrinologie Sexulle de la Pêriode Perinatale.* Forest, M.G., and Bertrand, J., eds. INSERM 32:407-420.

Larramendi, L.M.H. (1969): Analysis of synaptogenesis in the cerebellum of the mouse. *In: Neurobiology of Cerebellar Evolution and Development.* Llinás, R., ed. Chicago: American Medical Association, pp. 803-844.

Larsson, K., Sodersten, P., and Beyer, C. (1973): Sexual behavior in male rats treated with estrogen in combination with dihydrotestosterone. *Horm. Behav.* 4:289-299.

Laskowski, W. (1953): Reaktionen der primären and sekundaren Geshlechtsmerkmale von *Platypoecilus variatus* (Male heterogamet) und *Platypoecilus maculatus* (male hormogamet) auf Sexualhormone. *Arch. Entwicklungmech. Organ.* 146:(2)137-182.

Lassig, B.R. (1977): Socioecological strategies adopted by obligate coral dwelling fishes. *In: Proceedings of the Third International Coral Reef Symposium*, pp.565-570.

Lee, C.T. and Griffo, W. (1973): Early androgenization and aggression pheromone in inbred mice. *Horm. Behav.* 4:181-189.

Lee, R.B. (1965): Subsistence ecology of !Kung Bushmen. Doctoral Dissertation, University of California, Berkeley.

Lee, R.B. and DeVore, I., eds. (1968): *Man the Hunter.* Chicago: University of Chicago Press.

Lee, R.B. and DeVore, I., eds. (1976): *Kalahari Hunter-Gatherers.* Cambridge: Cambridge University Press.

Lehrman, D.S. (1964): The reproductive behavior of ring doves. *Sci. Am.* 211:48-54.

Leifer, A.D. (1970): Effects of early, temporary mother-infant separation on later maternal behavior in humans. Doctoral Dissertation, Stanford University, Stanford, CA.

Lenard, L. (1977): Sex-dependent body weight loss after bilateral 6-hydroxydopamine injection into the globus pallidus. *Brain Res.* 128:559-568.

Lenard, L., Sarkasian, J., and Szabo, I. (1975): Sex-dependent survival of rats after bilateral pallidal lesions. *Physiol. Behav.* 15:389-397.

Lentz, F.E., Jr., Pool, G.L., and Milner, J.S. (1978): Effects of ovariectomy and hormone replacement on DRL behavior in the rat. *Physiol. Behav.* 20:477-480.

Leonard, S. (1939): Induction of singing in female canaries by injections of male hormone. *Proc. Soc. Exp. Biol. Med.* 41:229-230.

Leutenegger, W. (1978): Scaling of sexual dimorphism in body size and breeding system in primates. *Nature* 272:610-611.

Levine, S. and Mullins, R., Jr. (1964): Estrogen administered neonatally affects adult sexual behavior in male and female rats. *Science* 144:185-187.

Lewis, M. and Rosenblum, L., eds. (1974): *The Effect of the Infant on Its Caregiver.* New York: John Wiley and Sons. Inc.

Lieberburg, I., Krey, L.C., and McEwen, B.S. (1979): Sex differences in serum testosterone and in exchangeable brain cell nuclear estradiol during the neonatal period in rats. *Brain Res.* (In press)

Lieberburg, I. and McEwen, B.S. (1975). Estradiol-17 β: a metabolite of testosterone recovered in cell nuclei from limbic areas of neonatal rat brains. *Brain Res.* 85:165-170.

Lieberburg, I. and McEwen, B.S. (1977): Brain cell nuclear retention of testosterone metabolites, 5α-dihydrotestosterone and estradiol-17β, in adult rats, *Endocrinology,* 100:588-597.

Lieberburg, I., Maclusky, N.J., and McEwen, B.S. (1977a): 5α-Dihydrotestosterone (DHT) receptors in rat brain and pituitary cell nuclei. *Endocrinology* 100:598-607.

Lieberburg, I. Wallach, G., and McEwen, B.S. (1977b): The effect of an inhibitor of aromatization (1, 4, 6-androstatriene-3,17-dione) and an anti-estrogen (CI-628) on in vivo formed testosterone metabolites recovered from neonatal rat brain tissues and purified cell nuclei. Implications for sexual differentiation of the rat brain. *Brain Res.* 128:176-181.

Lieblich, I., Isseroff, A., and Phillips, A.G. (1974): Developmental and hormonal aspects of increased emotionality produced by septal lesions in male rats: A parametric study of the effects of early castration. *Physiol. Behav.* 12-45-53.

Lill, A. (1974): Sexual behavior of the lek-forming white-bearded manakin *(Manacus manacus trinitatis* Hartert. *Z. Tiepsychol.* 36:1-36.

Lill, A. (1976): Lek behavior in the golden-headed manakin, *Pipra erythrocephala,* in Trinidad. *Fortschr. Verhaltensforsch.* 18:1-84.

Lindburg, D.G. (1971): The rhesus monkey in northern India: An ecological and behavioral study. *In: Primate Behavior: Developments in Field and Laboratory Research, Vol. 2.* New York: Academic Press, pp. 1-106.

Litteria, M. (1973): Inhibitory action of neonatal androgenization on the incorporation of (^{3}H)-lysine in specific hypothalamic nuclei of the adult female rat. *Exp. Neurol.* 41:395-401.

Litteria, M. and Thorner, M.W. (1974a): Inhibition in the incorporation of (^{3}H)-lysine in the Purkinje cells of the adult female rat after neonatal androgenization. *Brain Res.* 69:170-173.

Litteria, M. and Thorner, M.W. (1974b): Inhibitory effect of neonatal estrogenization on the incorporation of (^{3}H)-lysine in the Purkinje cells of the adult male and female rat. *Brain Res.* 80:152-154.

Litteria, M. and Thorner, M.W. (1975): Inhibitory action of neonatal estrogenization on the incorporation of (^{3}H)-lysine into proteins of specific hypothalamic nuclei in the adult, male rat. *Brain Res.* 90: 175-180.

Lloyd, T. and Weisz, J. (1978): Direct inhibition of tyrosine hydroxylase activity by catechol estrogens. *J. Biol. Chem.* 253:4841-4843.

Lloyd, T. and Weisz, J., and Breakefield, X. O. (1978): The catechol estrogen, 2-hydroxy-estradiol, inhibits catechol-*O*-methyltransferase activity in neuroblastoma cells. *J. Neurochem.* 31:245-250.

Lofts, B. and Murton, R.K. (1973): Reproduction in birds. *In: Avian Biology, Vol. 3.* Farner, D.S. and King, J.R., eds. New York: Academic Press, pp. 1-107.

Lording, D.W. and De Kretser, D.M. (1972): Comparative ultrastructural and histochemical studies of the interstitial cells of the rat testis during fetal and postnatal development. *J. Reprod. Fertil.* 29:261-269.

Lorens, S.A. and Kondo, C.Y. (1971): Differences in the consummatory and operant behaviors of male and female septal rats. *Physiol. Behav.* 6:487-491.

Lorenz, K. (1941): Vergleichende Bewegungsstudien an Anatinen. *J. Ornithol.* 89 (Suppl. 3): 194-293.

Lowenthal, M.F. (1975): Psychosocial variations across the adult life course: Frontiers for research and policy. *Gerontologist* 15:6-12.

Lowenthal, M., Thurnher, M., and Chiriboga, D. (1975): *Four Stages of Life: A Comparative Study of Men and Women Facing Transitions.* San Francisco: Jossey-Bass, Inc.

Lumia, A.R., Westervelt, M.O., and Rieder, C.A. (1975): Effects of olfactory bulb ablation and androgen on marking and agonistic behavior in male Mongolian gerbils, *Meriones unguiculatus. J. Comp. Physiol. Psychol.* 89:1091-1099.

Lund, J.S. and Lund, R. (1972): The effects of varying periods of visual deprivation on synaptogenesis in the superior colliculus of the rat. *Brain Res.* 42:21-32.

Luttge, W.G. (1975): Effects of antiestrogens on testosterone stimulated male sexual behavior and peripheral target tissues in the castrate male rat. *Physiol. Behav.* 14:839-846.

Luttge, W.G. and Hall, N.R. (1973a): Androgen-induced agonistic behavior in castrate male Swiss-Webster mice: comparison of four naturally occurring androgens. *Behav. Biol.* 8:725-732.

Luttge, W.G. and Hall, N.R. (1973b): Differential effectiveness of testosterone and its metabolites in the induction of male sexual behavior in two strains of albino mice. *Horm. Behav.* 4:31-43.

Luttge, W.G., Hall, N.R., and Wallis, C.J. (1974): Studies on the neuroendocrine, somatic and behavioral effectiveness of testosterone and its 5α-reduced metabolites in Swiss-Webster mice. *Physiol. Behav.* 13:553-561.

Luttge, W.G., Hall, N.R., Wallis, C.J., and Campbell, J.C. (1975): Stimulation of male and female sexual behavior in gonadectomized rats with estrogen and androgen therapy and its inhibition with concurrent anti-hormone therapy. *Physiol. Behav.* 14:65-73.

Luttge, W.G. and Whalen, R.E. (1970): Dihydrotestosterone, androstenedione, testosterone: comparative effectiveness in masculinizing and defeminizing reproductive systems in male and female rats. *Horm. Behav.* 1:265-281.

McCauley, E. and Ehrhardt, A.A. (1976): Female sexual response. Hormonal and behavioral interactions. *Primary Care* 3:455-476.

McDonald, R., Beyer, C., Newton, F., Brien, B., Baker, R., Tan, H.S., Sampson, C., Kitching, P., Greenhill, R., and Pritchard, D. (1970): Failure of 5α-dihydrotestosterone to initiate sexual behavior in the castrated male rat. *Nature* 227:964-965.

McDonald, P.G. and Doughty, C. (1972): Comparison of the effect of neonatal administration of testosterone and dihydrotestosterone in the female rat. *J. Reprod. Fertil.* 30:55-62.

McDonald, P.G. and Doughty, C. (1972): Inhibition of androgen-sterilization in the female rat by administration of an antioestrogen. *J. Endocrinol.* 55:455-456.

McEwen, B.S. (1976): Endocrine effects on the brain and their relationship to behavior. *In: Basic Neurochemistry.* Albers, W., et al., eds. Boston: Little, Brown and Co., pp. 737-764.

McEwen, B.S. (1976): Interactions between hormones and nerve tissue. *Sci. Am.* 235:48-58.

McEwen, B.S. (1976): Steroid hormone receptors in developing and mature brain tissue. *In: Society for Neuroscience Symposia, Vol. I. Neurotransmitters, Hormones and Receptors: Novel Approaches.* Ferrendelli, J.A., McEwen, B.S., and Snyder, S.H., eds. Bethesda, MD: Society for Neuroscience, pp. 50-66.

McEwen, B.S. (1976): Steroid receptors in neuroendocrine tissues: topography, subcellular distribution, and functional implications. *In: Subcellular Mechanisms in Reproductive Neuroendocrinology.* Naftolin, S., Ryan, K.J., and Davies, J., eds. Amsterdam: Elsevier/North-Holland Biomedical Press, pp. 277-304.

McEwen, B.S., Lieberburg, I., Chaptal, C., and Krey, L.C. (1977): Aromatization: important for sexual differentiation of the neonatal rat brain. *Horm. Behav.* 9:249-263.

McEwen, B.S., Lieberburg, I., Maclusky, N., and Plapinger, L. (1976): Interactions of testosterone and estradiol with the neonatal rat brain: protective mechanism and possible relationship to sexual differentiation. *Ann. Biol. Anim. Biochim. Biophys.* 16 (3):471-478.

McEwen, B.S., Plapinger, L., Chaptal, C., Gerlach, J., and Wallach, G. (1975): Role of fetoneonatal estrogen binding proteins in the associations of estrogen with neonatal brain cell nuclear receptors. *Brain Res.* 96:400-406.

McGill, T.E. (1970): Genetic analysis of male and sexual behavior. *In: Contributions to Behavior-Genetic Analysis. The Mouse as a Prototype.* Lindzey, G. and Thiessen, D.D., eds. New York: Appleton-Century-Crofts, pp. 57-88.

McGill, T.E., Albelda, S.M., Bible, H.H., and Williams, C.L. (1976): Inhibition of the ejaculatory reflex in B6D2F mice by testosterone propionate. *Behav. Biol.* 16:373-378.

McGill, T.E. and Manning, A. (1976): Genotype and retention of the ejaculatory reflex in castrated male mice. *Anim. Behav.* 24:507-518.

McGill, T. E. and Tucker, G.R. (1964): Genotype and sex drive in intact and castrated male mice. *Science* 145:514-515.

Machado-Magalhaes, H. and de Araujo-Carlini, E.L. (1974): Effects of perinatal testosterone treatment on body weight, open field behavior and Lashley III maze performance. *Acta Physiol. Lat. Am.* 24:317-327.

Maclusky, N.J., Chaptal, C., Lieberburg, I., and McEwen, B.S. (1976): Properties and subcellular inter-relationships of the presumptive estrogen receptor macromolecules in the brains of neonatal and prepubertal female rats. *Brain Res.* 114:158-165.

Maclusky, N.J., Chaptal, C., and McEwen, B.S. (1975): Postnatal ontogeny of cytoplasmic and nuclear estrogen-specific binding in the brain and pituitary of the rat. *In: Neuroscience Abstracts, Vol. 1.* (Fifth Annual Meeting of the Society for Neuroscience, New York City, Nov. 2-6, 1975.) P. 439.

Maclusky, N.J., Lieberburg, I., and McEwen, B.S. (1979): The development of estrogen receptor systems in the rat brain: gestational time of origin and perinatal development. *Brain Res.* (In press)

McNemar, Q. and Stone, C.P. (1932): The sex difference in rats on three learning tasks. *J. Comp. Psychol.* 14:171-180.

Madden, J.D., Walsh, P.C., MacDonald, P.C., and Wilson, J.D. (1975): Clinical and endocrinologic characterization of a patient with the syndrome of incomplete testicular feminization. *J. Clin. Endocrinol. Metab.* 40: 751-760.

Manning, A. (1967): The control of sexual receptivity in female *Drosophila. Anim. Behav.* 15:239-250.

Manning, A. (1975): Behaviour genetics and the study of behavioural evolution. *In: Function and Evolution in Behaviour. Essays in Honour of Professor Niko Tinbergen, F.R.S.* Baerends, G., Beer, C., and Manning, A., eds. London: Oxford University Press, pp. 71-91.

Manning, A. (1976): The place of genetics in the study of behaviour. *In: Growing Points in Ethology.* Bateson, P.P.G. and Hinde, R.A., eds. Cambirdge: Cambridge University Press, pp. 327-343.

Manning, A. and McGill, T.E. (1974): Neonatal androgen and sexual behavior in female house mice. *Horm. Behav.* 5:19-31.

Manning, A. and Thompson, M.L. (1976): Postcastration retention of sexual behaviour in the male BDF_1 mouse: The role of experience. *Anim. Behav.* 24:523-533.

Marcus, D.S., Schuler, H., Boccella, L., Zivic, W., and Josimovich, J.B. (1977): New techniques of injection of estradiol into preoptic-anterior hypothalamic area of newborn rats: technique limiting diffusion and duration, with preliminary results on postpubertal block of ovulation. *Endocrinology* 100:862-872.

Marić, D., Tadić, R., and Miline, R. (1974): The influence of gonads on the functional development of the hypothalamo-hypophysial system of the male rat. *Neuroendocrinology* 15: 92-98.

Marks, H.E., Fargason, B.D., and Hobbs, S.H. (1972): Reactivity to aversive stimuli as a function of alterations in body weight in normal and gonadectomized female rats. *Physiol. Behav.* 9:539-544.

Marks, H.E. and Hobbs, S.H. (1972): Changes in stimulus reactivity following gonadectomy in male and female rats of different ages. *Physiol. Behav.* 8:1113-1119.

Marler, P. (1956): Behaviour of the chaffinch, *Fringilla coelebs. Behaviour Suppl.* 5:1-84.

Marler, P. and Hamilton, W.J., III. (1966): *Mechanisms of Animal Behavior.* New York: John Wiley and Sons. Inc.

Marmor, J. and Green, R. (1977): Homosexual behavior. *In: Handbook of Sexology.* Money, J. and Musaph, H., eds. Amsterdam: Excerpta Medica, pp. 1051-1068.

Martinez-Vargas, M.C., Gibson, D.B., Sar, M., and Stumpf, W.E. (1975): Estrogen target sites in the brain of the chick embryo. *Science* 190:1307-1308.

Martini, L. (1976): Androgen reduction by neuroendocrine tissues: physiological significance. *In: Subcellular Mechanisms in Reproductive Neuroendocrinology.* Naftolin, F., Ryan, K.T., and Davis, J., eds. Amsterdam: Elsevier/North-Holland Biomedical Press, pp. 327-345.

Martins, T. and Valle, S.R. (1948): Hormonal regulation of the micturational behavior of the dog. *J. Comp. Physiol. Psychol.* 41:301-311.

Martucci, C. and Fishman, J. (1976): Uterine estrogen receptor of catecholestrogens and of estetrol (1, 3, 5 (10)-estratriene-3, 15 alpha, 16 alpha, 17 beta-tetrol). *Steroids* 27:325-333.

Masica, D.N., Money, J., and Ehrhardt, A.A. (1971): Fetal feminization and female gender identity in the testicular feminizing syndrome of androgen insensitivity. *Arch. Sex. Behav.* 1:131-142.

Mason, W.A. (1978): Ontogeny of social systems. *In: Recent Advances in Primatology, Vol. 1. Behaviour.* Chivers, D.J. and Herbert, J., eds. London: Academic Press, pp. 5-14.

Matsumoto, A. and Arai, Y. (1976): Effect of estrogen on early postnatal development of synaptic formation in the hypothalamic arcuate nucleus of female rats. *Neurosci. Lett.* 2:79-82.

Maurer, R.A. and Woolley, D.E. (1974): Demonstration of nuclear ^{3}H-estradiol binding in hypothalamus and amygdala of female, androgenized-female, and male rats. *Neuroendocrinology* 16:137-147.

Meijs-Roelofs, H.M.A., Uilenbroek, J.T., Jong, F.H. de, and Welschen, R. (1973): Plasma oestradiol-17 beta and its relationship to serum follicle-stimulating hormone in immature female rats. *J. Endocrinol.* 59:295-304.

Merchant-Larios, H. (1976): The onset of testicular differentiation in the rat: An ultrastructural study. *Am. J. Anat.* 145:319-329.

Meusy-Dessolle, N. (1974): Evolution de taux de testostérone plasmatique au cours de la vie foetale chez le porc domestique. *C.R. Acad. Sci. D* 278:1257-1260.

Meyer-Bahlburg, H.F.L. (1974): Aggression, androgens, and XYY syndrome. *In: Sex Differences in Behavior.* Friedman, R.C., Richart, R.M., and Vande Wiele, R.L., eds. New York: John Wiley and Sons, pp. 433-453.

Meyer-Bahlburg, H.F.L. (1977): Sex hormones and male homosexuality in comparative perspective. *Arch. Sex. Behav.* 6:297-326.

Meyer-Bahlburg, H.F.L., Grisanti, G.C., and Ehrhardt, A.A. (1977): Prenatal effects of sex hormones on human male behavior: medroxyprogesterone acetate (MPA). *Psychoneuroendocrinology* 2:383-390.

Milin, B. and Roy, A.K. (1973): Androgen "receptor" in rat liver: cytosol "receptor" deficiency in pseudohermaphrodite male rats. *Nature New Biol.* 242:248-250.

Millar, R., and Fairall, N. (1976): Hypothalamic, pituitary and gonadal hormone production in relation to nutrition in the male hyrax *(Procavia capensis). J. Reprod. Fertil.* 47:339-341.

Miller, A.E. (1970:) Effects of limited food consumption on body weight, locomotor activity and testis size of the Gambel's white-crowned sparrow (*Zonotrichia leucophrys gambelii*). Master's Thesis, San Jose State College, California.

Miller, R.A. (1938): Spermatogenesis in a sex-reversed female and in normal males of the domestic fowl. *Anat. Rec.* 70:155-189.

Mittwoch, U. (1970): How does the Y chromosome affect gonadal differentiation? *Phil Trans. Roy. Soc. B* 259:113-117.

Money, J. and Ehrhardt, A.A. (1972): *Man and Woman, Boy and Girl.* Baltimore: Johns Hopkins University Press.

Money, J. Ehrhardt, A.A. and Masica, D.N. (1968): Fetal feminization induced by androgen insensitivity in the testicular feminizing syndrome: effect on marriage and maternalism. *Johns Hopkins Med. J.* 123:105-114.

Money, J. and Schwartz, M. (1977): Dating, romantic and nonromantic friendship, sexuality in 17 early-treated AG females, aged 16-25. *In: Congenital Adrenal Hyperplasia.* Lee, P.A., et. al., eds. Baltimore: University Park Press, pp. 419-431.

Money, J. and Schwartz, M. (1978): Biosocial determinants of gender identity differentiation and development. *In: Biological Determinants of Sexual Behavior.* Hutchinson, J.B., ed. New York: John Wiley and Sons, Inc., pp. 765-784.

Mongkonpunya, K., Lin, Y.C., Noden, P.A., Oxender, W.D. and Nafs, H.D. (1975): Androgens in the bovine fetus and dam. *Proc. Soc. Exp. Biol. Med.* 148:489-493.

Moore, R.J., Griffin, J.E., and Wilson, J.D. (1975): Diminished 5 alpha-reductase activity in extracts of fibroblasts cultured from patients with familial incomplete male pseudohermaphroditism, Type 2. *J. Biol. Chem.* 250:7168-7172.

Morest, D.K. (1969): The growth dendrites in the mammalian brain. *Z. Anat. Enteisklungsgesch.* 128:290-317.

Morrell, J.I., Kelley, D.B., and Pfaff, D.W. (1975): Sex steroid binding in the brains of vertebrates. *In: Brain-Endocrine Interaction II.* Knigge, K.M. et al., eds. Basel: S. Karger, pp. 230-256.

Morris, D. (1956): The function and causation of courtship ceremonies. *In: L'Instinct dans le Comportement des Animaux et de l'Homme.* Fondation Singer-Polignac. Paris: Masson et Cie, pp. 261-286.

Morris, D. (1957): "Typical intensity" and its relation to the problem of ritualization. *Behaviour* 9:1-12.

Moynihan, M. (1955): Some aspects of reproductive behavior in the black-headed gull *(Larus ridibundus ridibundus* L.) and related species. *Behaviour Suppl.* 4:1-201.

Mullins, R.F., Jr. and Levine, S. (1968): Hormonal determinants during infancy of adult sexual behavior in the female rat. *Physiol. Behav.* 3:333-338.

Murgita, R.A. and Tomasi, T.B. (1975): Suppression of the immune response by alpha-fetoprotein on the primary and secondary antibody response. *J. Exp. Med.* 141:269-286.

Nadler, R.D. (1968): Masculinization of female rats by intracranial implantation of androgen in infancy. *J. Comp. Physiol. Psychol.* 66:157-167.

Nadler, R.D. (1969): Differentiation of the capacity for male sexual behavior in the rat. *Horm. Behav.* 1:53-63.

Nadler, R.D. (1972): Intrahypothalamic locus for induction of androgen sterilization in neonatal female rats. *Neuroendocrinology* 9:349-357.

Nadler, R.D. (1973): Further evidence on the intrahypothalamic locus for androgenization of female rats. *Neuroendocrinology* 12:110-119.

Naess, O., Haug, E., Attramadal, A., Aakvaag, A., Hansson, V., and French, F. (1976): Androgen receptors in the anterior pituitary and central nervous system of the androgen "insensitive" (Tfm) rat: correlation between receptor binding and effects of androgens on gonadotropin secretion. *Endocrinology* 99:1295-1303.

Naftolin, F., Morishita, H., Davies, I.J., Todd, R., Ryan, K.J. (1975a): 2-Hydroxyestrone induced rise in serum luteinizing hormone in the immature male rat. *Biochem. Biophys. Res. Commun.* 64:905-910.

Naftolin, F., Ryan, K.J., Davies, I.J., Reddy, V.V., Flores, F., Petro, Z., Kuhn, M., White, R.J., Takaoka, Y., and Wolin, L. (1975b): The formation of estrogens by central neuroendocrine tissues. *Rec. Prog. Horm. Res.* 31:295-319.

Naftolin, F., Ryan, K.J., and Petro, Z. (1971): Aromatization of androstenedione by the diencephalon. *J. Clin. Endocrinol. Metab.* 33:368-370.

Nakai, T., Kigawa, T., and Sakamoto, S. (1971): ^{3}H-Leucine uptake of hypothalamic nuclei in fetal male rats and its fluctuation after castration. *Endocrinol. Jpn.* 18:353-357.

Nance, D.M. (1976): Sex differences in the hypothalamic regulation of feeding behavior. *In: Advances in Psychobiology, Vol. 3.* Riesen, A.H. and Thompson, R.F., eds. New York: John Wiley and Sons, pp. 75-123.

Nance, D.M. and Gorski, R.A. (1975): Neurohormonal determinants of sex differences in the hypothalamic regulation of feeding behavior and body weight in the rat. *Pharmacol. Biochem. Behav. (Suppl. 1)* 3:155-162.

Nance, D.M., Phelps, C., Shryne, J.E., and Gorski, R.A. (1977): Alterations by estrogen and hypothyroidism in the effects of septal leisions on lordosis behavior of male rats. *Brain Res. Bull.* 2:49-53.

Nance, D.M., Shryne, J., and Gorski, R.A. (1975): Facilitation of female sexual behavior in male rats by septal lesions: An interaction with estrogen. *Horm. Behav.* 6:289-299.

Napoli, A.M. and Gerall, A.A. (1970): Effect of estrogen and anti-estrogen on reproductive function in neonatally androgenized female rats. *Endocrinology* 87:1330-1337.

Narbaitz, R. and Adler, R. (1967): Submicroscopical aspects in the differentiation of rat fetal Leydig cells. *Acta Physiol. Lat. Am.* 17:286-291.

Neill, J.D. (1972): Sexual differences in the hypothalamic regulation of prolactin secretion. *Endocrinology* 90:1154-1159.

Nelson, J.B. (1965): The behaviour of the Gannet. *Br. Birds* 58:233-288.

Neumann, F. and Steinbeck, H. (1974): Differentiation of neural centers. *In: Handbook of Experimental Pharmacology, Vol. 35. Androgens II and Antiandrogens.* Eichler, O., Farah, A., Herken, H., and Welch, A.D., eds. Berlin: Springer-Verlag, pp. 382-399.

Newton, N. (1963): Emotions of pregnancy. *Clin. Obstet. Gynecol.* 6:639-668.

Nicolai, J. (1964): Der Brutparasitismus der Viduinen als ethologisches Problem. Prägungsphänomene als Faktoren der Rassen- und Artbildung. *Z. Tierpsychol.* 21:129-204.

Niemi, M. and Ikonen, M. (1961): Steroid-3β-ol-dehydrogenase activity in foetal Leydig's cells. *Nature* 189:592-593.

Niemi, M. and Ikonen, M. (1963): Histochemistry of the Leydig cells in the postnatal prepubertal testis of the rat. *Endocrinology* 72:443-448.

Noble, R. (1974): Estrogen plus androgen induced mounting in adult female hamsters. *Horm. Behav.* 5:227-234.

Noble, R.G. (1977): Mounting in female hamsters: Effects of different hormone regimens. *Physiol. Behav.* 19:519-526.

Nottebohm, F. (1968): Auditory experience and song development in the chaffinch, *Fringilla coelebs. Ibis* 110:549-568.

Nottebohm, F. (1969): The "critical period" for song learning. *Ibis* 111:386-387.

Nottebohm, F. (1972): The origins of vocal learning. *Am. Nat.* 105:116-140.

Nottebohm, F. (1975): Vocal behavior in birds. *In: Avian Biology, Vol. 5.* Farner, D.S. and King, J.R., eds. New York: Academic Press. pp. 287-332.

Nottebohm, F. (1979): Testosterone triggers growth of brain vocal control areas in adult female canaries. *Science* (In press)

Nottebohm, F. and Arnold, A.P. (1976): Sexual dimorphism in vocal control areas of the songbird brain. *Science* 194:211-213.

Nottebohm, F. and Nottebohm, M. (1971): Vocalizations and breeding behaviour of surgically deafened ring doves (*Streptopelia risoria*). *Anim. Behav.* 19-313-327.

Nottebohm, F., Stokes, T.M., and Leonard, C.M. (1976): Central control of song in the canary, *Serinus canarius. J. Comp. Neurol.* 165:457-486.

Noumura, T., Weisz, J., and Lloyd, C.W. (1966): In vitro conversion of 7-^{3}H-progesterone to androgens in the rat testis during the second half of fetal life. *Endocrinology* 78:245-253.

Nucci, L.P. and Beach, F.A. (1971): Effects of prenatal androgen treatment on mating behavior in female hamsters. *Endocrinology* 88:1514-1515.

Nunez. E., Englemann, F., Benassayag, C., and Jayle, M.-F. (1971): Identification et purification préliminaire de la foeto-protiene liant les estrogenes dans le serum de rats nouveau-nes. *C.R. Acad. Sci. D* 173:831-834.

Ohno, S., Geller, L.N., and Young Lai, E.V. (1974): Tfm mutation and masculinization versus feminization of the mouse central nervous system. *Cell* 3:237-244.

Orcutt, F.S. (1971): Effects of oestrogen on the differentiation of some reproductive behaviours in male pigons (*Columba livia*). *Anim. Behav.* 19:277-286.

Ortiz, E., Price, D., and Zaaijer, J.J.P. (1966): Organ culture studies of hormone secretion in endocrine glands of fetal guinea pigs. II. Secretion of androgenic hormone in adrenals and testes during early stages of development. *Proc. Kon. Nederl. Akad. Wet. (Biol. Med.)* 69:400-408.

Ozon, R. (1965): Mise en évidence d'hormones stéroides oestrogènes dans le sang de la poule adulte et chez l'embryon de poulet. *C.R.Acad.Sci.D* 261:5664-5666.

Palade, G.E., (1955): A small particulate component of the cytoplasm. *J. Biophys. Biochem. Cytol.* 1:59-68.

Paré, W.P. (1969): Age, sex, and strain differences in the aversive threshold to grid shock in the rat. *J. Comp. Physiol. Psychol.* 69:214-218.

Parker, J.E. and Arscott, G.H. (1964): Energy intake and fertility of male chickens. *J. Nutr.* 82: 183-187.

Parlee, M.A. (1975): Psychological aspects of menstruation, childbirth and menopause: an overview with suggestions for further research. Paper presented at Conference on New Directions for Research on Women, Madison, WI, May 31-June 2.

Parmelee, D.F. (1970): Breeding behavior of the sanderling in the Canadian high Arctic. *Living Bird* 9:97-146.

Parmelee, D.F. and Payne, R.B. (1973): On multiple broods and the breeding strategy of arctic sanderlings. *Ibis* 11:218-226.

Parnavelas, J.G., Globus, A., and Kaups, P. (1973): Changes in lateral geniculate neurons of rats as a result of continuous exposure to light. *Nature New Biol.* 245:287-288.

Parrot, R.F. (1975): Aromatizable and 5α-reduced androgens: differentiation between central and peripheral effects on male rat sexual behavior. *Horm. Behav.* 6:99-108.

Parrot, R.F. (1975): Stimulation of sexual behavior in male and female rats with the synthetic androgen, 17β-hydroxyoestra-4-en-3-one (19-nortestosterone). *J. Endocrinol.* 65:285-286.

Parvizi, N. and Ellendorf, F. (1975): 2-hydroxy-oestradiol-17β as a possible link in steroid brain interaction. *Nature* 256:59-60.

Paup, D.C., Coniglio, L.P., and Clemens, L.G. (1972): Masculinization of the female golden hamster by neonatal treatment with androgen or estrogen. *Horm. Behav.* 3:123-131.

Paup, D.C., Coniglio, L.P., and Clemens, L.G. (1974): Hormonal determinants in the development of masculine and feminine behavior in the female hamster. *Behav. Biol.* 10:353-363.

Paup, D.C., Mennin, S.P., and Gorski, R.A. (1975): Androgen- and estrogen-induced copulatory behavior and inhibition of luteinizing hormone (LH) secretion in the male rat. *Horm. Behav.* 6:35-46.

Payne, A.H. and Jaffe, R.B. (1975): Androgen formation from pregnenolone sulfate by fetal, neonatal, prepubertal and adult human testes. *J. Clin Endocrinol. Metab.* 40:102-107.

Payne, A.H., Kelch, R.P., Murono, E.P., and Kerlan, J.T. (1977): Hypothalamic, pituitary and testicular function during sexual maturation of the male rat. *J. Endocrinol.* 72:17-26.

Payne, A.P. (1973): A comparison of the aggressive behaviour of isolated intact and castrated male golden hamsters towards intruders introduced into the home cage. *Physiol. Behav.* 10: 629-631.

Payne, A.P. and Swanson, H.H. (1971a): The effect of castration and ovarian implantation on aggressive behavior of male hamsters. *J. Endocrinol.* 51:217-218.

Payne, A.P. and Swanson, H.H. (1971b): Hormonal control of aggressive dominance in the female hamster. *Physiol. Behav.* 5:355-357.

Payne, A.P. and Swanson, H.H. (1972a): The effect of sex hormones on the aggressive behavior of the female golden hamster (*Mesocricetus auratus* Waterhouse). *Anim. Behav.* 20:782-787.

Payne, A.P. and Swanson, H.H. (1972b): The effect of sex hormones on the agonistic behavior of the male golden hamster (*Mesocricetus auratus* Waterhouse). *Physiol. Behav.* 8:687-691.

Payne, A.P. and Swanson, H.H. (1972c): Neonatal androgenization and aggression in the male golden hamster. *Nature* 239:282-283.

Payne, R.B. (1973): Vocal mimicry of the paradise whydahs (*Vidua*) and response of female whydahs to the songs of their hosts (*Pytilia*) and their mimics. *Anim. Behav.* 21:762-771.

Peters, P.J., Bronson, F.H., and Whitsett, J.M. (1972): Neonatal castration and intermale aggression in mice. *Physiol. Behav.* 8:265-268.

Petrusz, P. and Flerko, B. (1968): Effect of ovariectomy and oestrogen administration on the pituitary and uterine weight in androgen-sterilized rats. *Acta Biol. Acad. Sci. Hung.* 19 159-162.

Petrusz, P. and Nagy, E. (1967): On the mechanism of sexual differentiation of the hypothalamus. Decreased hypothalamic oestrogen sensitivity in androgen-sterilized female rats. *Acta Biol. Acad. Sci. Hung.* 18:21-26.

Pfaff, D.W. (1966): Morphological changes in the brains of adult male rats after neonatal castration. *J. Endocrinol.* 36:415-416.

Pfaff, D. (1970): Nature of sex hormone effects on rat sex behavior. Specificity of effects and individual patterns of response. *J. Comp. Physiol. Psychol.* 73:349-358.

Pfaff, D.W. and Zigmond, R.E. (1971): Neonatal androgen effects on sexual and non-sexual behavior of adult rats tested under various hormone regimes. *Neuroendocrinology* 7: 129-145.

Phelps, C.P. and Sawyer, C.H. (1976): Postnatal thyroxine modifies effects of early androgen on lordosis. *Horm. Behav.* 7:331-340.

Phillips, A.G. and Deol, G. (1973): Neonatal gonadal hormone manipulation and emotionality following septal lesions in weanling rats. *Brain Res.* 60:55-64.

Phillips, A.G. and Lieblich, I. (1972): Developmental and hormonal aspects of hyperemotionality produced by septal lesions in male rats. *Physiol. Behav.* 9:237-242.

Phoenix, C.H. (1974): Effects of dihydrotestosterone on sexual behavior of castrated male rhesus monkeys. *Physiol. Behav.* 12:1045-1055.

Phoenix, C.H., Goy, R.W., Gerall, A.A., and Young, W.C. (1959): Organizational action of prenatally administered testosterone propionate on the tissues mediating behavior in the female guinea pig. *Endocrinology* 65:369-382.

Phoenix, C.H., Goy, R.W., and Resko, J.A. (1968): Psychosexual differentiation as a function of androgenic stimulation. *In: Perspectives in Reproduction and Sexual Behavior.* Diamond, M., ed. Bloomington: Indiana University Press, pp. 33-49.

Picon, R. (1976): Testosterone secretion by foetal rat testes *in vitro*. *J. Endocrinol.* 71: 231-238.

Pirani, B.B., Pairaudeau, N., Doran, T.A., Wong, P.Y., and Gardner, H.A. (1977): Amniotic fluid testosterone in the prenatal determination of fetal sex. *Am. J. Obstet. Gynecol.* 129: 518-520.

Plapinger, L. and McEwen, B.S. (1973): Ontogeny of estradiol-binding sites in rat brain. I. Appearance of presumptive adult receptors in cytosol and nuclei. *Endocrinology* 93:1119-1128.

Plapinger, L. and McEwen, B.S. (1975): Immunochemical comparison of estradiol-binding macromolecules in perinatal rat brain cytosol and serum. *Steroids* 26:255-265.

Plapinger, L. and McEwen, B.S. (1978): Gonadal steriod-brain interactions in sexual differentiation. *In: Biological Determinants of Sexual Behavior.* Hutchison, J., ed. New York: John Wiley and Sons.

Plapinger, L., McEwen, B.S., and Clemens, L.E. (1973): Ontogeny of estradiol-binding sites in rat brain. II. Characteristics of a neonatal binding macromolecule. *Endocrinology* 93: 1129-1139.

Pollak, E.I. and Sachs, B.D. (1975): Masculine sexual behavior and morphology: paradoxical effects of perinatal androgen treatment in male and female rats. *Behav. Biol.* 13:401-411.

Pomerantz, D.K. and Nalbandov, A.V. (1975): Androgen level in the sheep fetus during gestation. *Proc. Soc. Exp. Biol. Med.* 149:413-416.

Popper, D. and Fishelson, L. (1973): Ecology and behavior of *Anthias squamipinnis* (Peters, 1855) (Anthibiae, teleostei) in the coral habitat of Eliat. *J. Exp. Zool.* 184:409-423.

Poulsen, H. (1951): Inheritance and learning in the song of the chaffinch (*Fringilla coelebs*). *Behaviour* 3:216-228.

Powell, D.A., Francis, J., and Schneiderman, N. (1971): The effect of castration, neonatal testosterone, and previous experience with fighting on shock-elicited aggression. *Commun. Behav. Biol.* 5:371-377.

Powley, T.L. and Keesey, R.E. (1970): Relationship of body weight to the lateral hypothalamic feeding syndrome. *J. Comp. Physiol. Psychol.* 70:25-36.

Presl, J., Pospisil, J., and Horsky, J. (1971): Autoradiographic localization of radioactivity in female rat neocortex after injection of tritiated estradiol. *Experientia* 27:465-467.

Prestige, M.C. (1970): Differentiation, degeneration and the role of the periphery: quantitative considerations. *In: The Neurosciences: Second Study Program.* Quarton, G.C., Melnechuk, T., and Schmitt, F.O., eds. New York: Rockefeller University Press, pp. 73-82.

Price, D., Ortiz, E. and Zaaijer, J.J.P. (1967): Organ culture studies of hormone secretion in endocrine glands of fetal guinea pigs. III. The relation of testicular hormone in sex differentiation of the reproductive ducts. *Anat. Rec.* 157:27-41.

Price, D. and Pannabecker, R. (1956): Organ culture studies of foetal rat reproductive tracts. *Ciba Found. Colloquia on Ageing* 2:3-17.

Pröve, E. (1974): Der Einflus von Kastration und Testosteronsubstitution auf das Sexualverhalten männlicher Zebrafinken. *J. Ornithol. 1.* 115:338-347.

Quadagno, D.M., Shryne, J., Anderson, C., and Gorski, R.A. (1972): Influence of gonadal hormones in social, sexual, emergence, and open field behavior in the rat, *Rattus norvegicus. Anim. Behav.* 20:732-740.

Raisman, G. (1974): Evidence for a sex difference in the neuropil of the rat preoptic area and its importance for the study of sexually dimorphic functions. *Assoc. Res. Nerv. Ment. Dis.* 52:42-51.

Raisman, G. and Field, P.M. (1971): Sexual dimorphism in the preoptic area of the rat. *Science* 173:731-733.

Raisman, G. and Field, P.M. (1973): Sexual dimorphism in the neuropil of the preoptic area of the rat and its dependence on neonatal androgen. *Brain Res.* 54:1-29.

Ramón y Cajal, S. (1955): *Histologie du Systême Nerveux de l'Homme et des Vêrtêbres, Vol. II.* Madrid: Consejo Superior de Investigacoines Cientificas, Instituto Ramón y Cajal.

Raynaud, J.P. (1973): Influence of rat estradiol binding plasma protein (EBP) on uterotrophic activity. *Steroids* 21:249-258.

Raynaud, J.P., Mercier-Bodard, C., and Baulieu, E.E. (1971): Rat estradiol binding plasma protein (EBP). *Steriods* 18:767-788.

Rebière, A. and Legrand, J. (1972): Données quantitatives sur la synaptogenèse dans le cervelet du rat normal et rendu hypothyroidien par le propylthiouracile. *C.R. Acad. Sci. D* 274: 3581-3584.

Reddy, V.V.R., Naftolin, F., and Ryan, K.J. (1974): Conversion of androstenedione to estrone by neural tissues from fetal and neonatal rats. *Endocrinology* 94:117-121.

Reier, P.J., Cullen, M.J., Froelich, J.S., et al. (1977): The ultrastructure of the developing medial preoptic nucleus in the postnatal rat. *Brain Res.* 122:415-436.

Rennie, P.S., Koat, A., and Bruchovsky, N. (1977): Androgenic regulation of acid phosphatase activity of rat ventral prostrate. *In: Program and Abstracts, Endocrine Society, Chicago, 1977.* Abstr. 58.

Resko, J.A. (1970): Androgen secretion by the fetal and neonatal rhesus monkey. *Endocrinology* 87:680-687.

Resko, J.A. (1974): The relationship between fetal hormones and the differentiation of the central nervous system in primates. *In: Reproductive Behavior.* Montagna, W. and Sadler, W.A., eds. New York: Plenum Press, pp. 211-222.

Resko, J.A. (1975): Fetal hormones and their effect on the differentiation of the central nervous system in primates. *Fed. Proc.* 34:1650-1655.

Resko, J.A., Feder, H.H., and Goy, R.W. (1968): Androgen concentrations in plasma and testes of developing rats. *J. Endocrinol.* 40:485-491.

Resko, J.A., Malley, A., Begley, D., and Hess, D.C. (1973): Radioimmunoassay of testosterone during fetal development of the rhesus monkey. *Endocrinology* 93:156-161.

Reyes, F.I., Boroditsky, R.S., Winter, J.S.D., and Faiman, C. (1974): Studies on human sexual development. II. Fetal and maternal serum gonadotropin and sex steroid concentration. *J. Clin. Metab.* 38:612-617.

Riddell, W.I., Galvani, P.F., and Foster, K.M. (1975): The role of escape-motivated behavior in aversive conditioning in rats and gerbils. *Behav. Biol.* 17:485-494.

Robel, R., Lasnitzki, I., and Baulieu, E.E. (1971): Hormone metabolism and action: testosterone and metabolites in prostrate organ culture. *Biochemie.* 53:81-96.

Robertson, D.R. (1972): Social control of sex reversal in a coral-reef fish. *Science* 177: 1007-1009.

Robinson, J.D., Judd, H.L., Young, P.E., Jones, W.W., and Yen, S.S. (1977): Amniotic fluid androgens and estrogens in midgestation. *J. Clin. Endocrinol. Metab.* 45:755-761.

Robson, K.S. and Moss, H.A. (1970): Patterns and determinants of maternal attachment. *J. Pediatr.* 77:976-985.

Rohde, W., Stahl, F., and Dörner, G. (1977): Plasma basal levels of FSH, LH and testosterone in homosexual men. *Endokrinologie* 70:241-248.

Rollins, B. and Cannon, K. (1974): Marital satisfaction over the family life cycle: a reevaluation *J. Marriage Fam.* 36:271-283.

Rollins, B. and Feldman, H. (1970): Marital satisfaction over the family life cycle. *J. Marriage Fam.* 32:20-28.

Roosen-Runge, E.C. and Anderson, D. (1959): The development of the interstitial cells in the testis of the albino rat. *Acta Anat.* 37:125-137.

Rossi, A.S. (1968): Transition to parenthood. *J. Marriage Fam.* 30:26-39.

Rossi, A.S. (1972: Family development in a changing world. *Am. J. Psychiatry* 128:1057-1066.

Rossi, A.S. (1973): Maternalism, sexuality, and the new feminism. *In: Contemporary Sexual Behavior: Critical Issues in the 1970s.* Zubin, J. and Money, J., eds. Baltimore: Johns Hopkins University Press, pp. 145-173.

Rossi, A.S.. (1977a): A biosocial perspective on parenting. *Daedalus.* 106(2):1-31.

Rossi, A.S. (1977b): Body time and social time: mood patterns by menstrual cycle phase and day of the week. *Soc. Sci. Res.* 6:273-308.

Rothstein, S.I. (1975): An experimental and teleonomic investigation of avian brood parasitism. *Condor* 77:250-271.

Rowell, T.E. (1966): Hierarchy in the organization of a captive baboon group. *Anim. Behav.* 14:430-443.

Rowell, T. (1972): *The Social Behavior of Monkeys.* Baltimore: Penguin Books, Inc.

Rowell, T. (1978): How female reproductive cycles affect interaction patterns in groups of patas monkeys. *In: Recent Advances in Primatology, Vol. 1 Behaviour.* Chivers, D.J. and Herbert, J., eds. London: Academic Press, pp. 489-490.

Roy, E.J., Maass, C.A., and Wade, G.N. (1977): Central action and a species comparison of the estrogenic effects of an antiestrogen on eating and body weight. *Physiol. Behav.* 18:137-140.

Roy, E.J. and Wade, G.N. (1975): Role of estrogens in androgen-induced spontaneous activity in male rats. *J. Comp. Physiol. Psychol.* 89:573-579.

Roy, E.J. and Wade, G.N. (1976): Estrogenic effects of an antiestrogen, MER-25, on eating and body weight in rats. *J. Comp. Physiol. Psychol.* 90:156-166.

Ruh, T.S. and Ruh, M.F. (1974): The effect of antiestrogens on the nuclear binding of the estrogen receptor. *Steroids* 24:209-224.

Ruiz-Marcos, A. and Valverde, F. (1969): The temporal evolution of the distribution of dendritic spines in the visual cortex of normal and dark raised mice. *Exp. Brain Res.* 8:284-294.

Rusak, B. and Zucker, I. (1975): Biological rhythms and animal behavior. *Ann. Rev. Psychol.* 26:137-171.

Sachs, B.D., Pollak, E.I., Krieger, M.A., and Barfield, R.J. (1973): Sexual behavior: Normal male patterning in androgenized female rats. *Science* 181:770-772.

Sadleir, R.M.F.S. (1969): *The Ecology of Reproduction in Wild and Domestic Mammals.* London: Methuen.

Salaman, D.F. (1974): The role of DNA, RNA and protein synthesis in sexual differentiation of the brain. *Prog. Brain Res.* 41:349-362.

Salaman, D.F. (1977): Effect of colchicine on androgen-induced sexual differentiation of the brain. *J. Endocrinol.* 72:54P-55P.

Salaman, D.F. and Birkett, S.I. (1974): Androgen-induced sexual differentiation of the brain is blocked by inhibitors of DNA and RNA synthesis. *Nature* 247:109-112.

Sanyal, M.K. and Villee, C.A. (1977): Stimulation of androgen biosynthesis in rat fetal testes *in vitro* by gonadotrophins. *Biol. Reprod.* 16:174-181.

Sayler, A. (1970): The effect of anti-androgens on aggressive behavior in the gerbil. *Physiol. Behav.* 5:667-671.

Schally, A.V., Arimura, A., and Kastin, A.J. (1973): Hypothalamic regulatory hormones. *Science* 179:341-350.

Schlegel, R.J., Farias, E., Russo, N.C., Moore, J.R., and Gardner, L.I. (1967): Structural changes in the fetal gonads and gonaducts during maturation of an enzyme, steroid 3β-ol dehydrogenase, in the gonads, adrenal cortex and placenta of fetal rats. *Endocrinology* 81:565-572.

Schultz, F.M. and Wilson, J.D. (1974): Virilization of the Wolffian duct in the rat fetus by various androgens. *Endocrinology* 94:979-986.

Schwartz, I.R., Pappas, G.D., and Purpura, D.P. (1968): Fine structure of neurons and synapses in the feline hippocampus during postnatal ontogenesis, *Exp. Neurol.* 22:394-407.

Schwartz, M. and Money, J. (1976): Athletics, dating, romance, friendships and sexuality in adrenogenital females, aged 16-26. International Congress of Sexology, Montreal Oct. 28-31, 1976. Abstr. 94.

Schwarzel, W.C., Kruggel, W.G., and Brodie, H.J. (1973): Study on the mechanism of estrogen biosynthesis. VII. The development of inhibitors of the enzyme system in human placenta. *Endocrinology* 92:866-880.

Scouten, C.W. (1972): Hormonal effects on avoidance in rats. Masters Thesis, North Dakota State University, Fargo.

Scouten, C.W., Groteleuschen, L.K., and Beatty, W.W. (1975): Androgens and the organization of sex differences in active avoidance behavior in the rat. *J. Comp. Physiol. Psychol.* 88: 264-270.

Selmanoff, M.K., Brodkin, L.D., Weiner, L.D., and Siiteri, P.K. (1977): Aromatization and 5α-reduction of androgens in discrete hypothalamic and limbic regions of the male and female rat. *Endocrinology* 101:841-848.

Selmanoff, M.K., Jumonville, J.E., Maxson, S.C., and Ginsburg, B.E. (1975): Evidence for a Y chromosomal contribution to an aggressive phenotype in inbred mice. *Nature* 253:529-530.

Shapiro, B.H. and Goldman, A.S. (1973): Feminine saccharin preference in the genetically androgen-insensitive male rat pseudohermaphrodite. *Horm. Behav.* 4:371-375.

Shapiro, B.H., Goldman, A.S., and Gustafsson, J.A. (1975): Masculine-like hypothalamic-pituitary axis in the androgen-insensitive genetically male rat pseudohermaphrodite. *Endocrinology* 97:487-492.

Shapiro, B.H., Goldman, A.S., Steinbeck, H.F., and Neumann, F. (1976): Is feminine differentiation of the brain hormonally determined? *Experientia* 42:650-651.

Shapiro, D.Y. (1977): Social organization and sex reversal of the coral reef fish *Anthias squamipinnis* (Peters). Ph.D. Dissertation, Gonville and Caius College, Cambridge University.

Sheridan, P.J., Sar, M., and Stumpf, W.E. (1974): Autoradiographic localization of ^{3}H-estradiol or its metabolites in the central nervous system of the developing rat. *Endocrinology* 94: 1386-1390.

Sheridan, P.J., Sar, M., and Stumpf, W.E. (1974): Interaction of exogenous steroids in the developing rat brain. *Endocrinology* 95:1749-1753.

Shoemaker, H.H. (1939): Effect of testosterone proprionate on the behavior of the female canary. *Proc. Soc. Exp. Biol. Med.* 41:299-302.

Short, R.V. (1970): The bovine freemartin: a new look at an old problem. *Phil. Trans. Roy. Soc. B* 259:141-147.

Short, R.V. (1974): Sexual differentiation in the brain of the sheep. *In: Endocrinologie Sexuelle de la Përiode Përinatale.* Forest, M.G. and Bertrand, J., eds. Paris: *INSERM* 32:121-142.

Slater, J. and Blizard, D.A. (1976): A reevaluation of the relation between estrogen and emotionality in female rats. *J. Comp. Physiol. Psychol.* 90:755-764.

Slob, A.K., Goy, R.W., and van der Werff ten Bosch, J.J. (1973): Sex differences in growth of guinea pigs and their modification by neonatal gonadectomy and prenatally administered androgen. *J. Endocrinol.* 58:11-19.

Slob, A.K. and van der Werff ten Bosch, J.J. (1975): Sex differences in body growth in the rat. *Physiol. Behav.* 14:353-361.

Smeaton, T.C., Arcondoulis, D.E., and Steele, P.A. (1975). The synthesis of testosterone and estradiol-17β by the gonads of neonatal rats *in vitro. Steroids* 26:181-192.

Snow, D.W. (1968): The singing assemblies of little hermits. *Living Bird* 7:47-55.

Södersten, P. (1973): Estrogen-activated sexual behavior in male rats. *Horm. Behav.* 4:247-256.

Södersten, P. (1974): Effects of an estrogen antagonist, MER-25, on mounting behavior and lordosis behavior in the female rat. *Horm. Behav.* 5:111-121.

Södersten, P. (1976): Lordosis behaviour in male, female and androgenized rats. *J. Endocrinol.* 70:409-420.

Soloff, M.S., Creange, J.E., and Potts, G.O. (1971): Unique estrogen-binding properties of rat pregnancy plasma. *Endocrinology* 88:427-432.

Southwick, C.H., ed. (1963): *Primate Social Behavior.* Princeton, N.J.: D. Van Nostrand Company, Inc.

Spanier, G., Lewis, R., and Cole, C. (1975): Marital adjustment over the family life cycle: the issue of curvilinearity. *J. Marriage Fam.* 37:263-275.

Stahl, F., Dörner, G., Ahrens, L., and Graudenz, G. (1976): Significantly decreased apparently free testosterone levels in plasma of male homosexuals. *Endokrinologie* 68:115-117.

Staudt, J. and Dörner, G. (1976): Structural changes in the medial and central amygdala of the male rat, following neonatal castration and androgen treatment. *Endokrinologie* 67:296-300.

Stern, D. (1974): Mother and infant at play: the dyadic interaction involving facial, vocal, and gaze behavior. *In: The Effect of the Infant on its Caregiver.* Lewis, M. and Rosenblum, L.A. eds. New York: John Wiley and Sons, Inc., pp. 187-213.

Stern, J.J. and Janowiak, P. (1973): No effect of neonatal estrogenic stimulation or hypophysectomy on spontaneous activity in female rats. *J. Comp. Physiol. Psychol.* 85:409-412.

Sternberger, L.A., Hardy, P.H., Cuculis, J.J., and Meyer, H.G. (1970): The unlabeled antibody-enzyme method of immunohistochemistry: Preparation and properties of soluble antigen-antibody complex (horseradish peroxidase-antiperoxidase) and its use in identification of spirochetes. *J. Histochem. Cytochem.* 18:315-333.

Stetson, M.H. and Watson-Whitmyre, M. (1976): Nucleus suprachiasmaticus: The biological clock in the hamster? *Science* 191:197-199.

Stewart, A.D., Manning, A., and Batty, J. (1979): Effects of the Y-chromosome in mice: a study of testis weight plasma testosterone and behaviour. *Heredity* (In press)

Stewart, J., Pottier, J., and Kaczender-Henrik, E. (1971): Male copulatory behavior in the female rat after perinatal treatment with an antiandrogenic steroid. *Horm. Behav.* 2:247-254.

Stewart, J., Skvarenina, A., and Pottier, J. (1975): Effects of neonatal androgens on open-field and maze learning in the prepubescent and adult rat. *Physiol. Behav.* 14:291-295.

Stinnakre, M.G. (1975): Période de sensibilité aux androgènes du canal de Wolff de foetus de rat. *Arch. Anat. Microsc. Morphol. Exp.* 64:45-59.

Studelska, D.R. and Beatty, W.W. (1976): Sex differences in the effects of neostriatal lesions on open-field and avoidance behavior in rats. Paper presented at the Annual Meeting of the Eastern Conference on Reproductive Behavior, Saratoga Springs, N.Y., June.

Studelska, D.R. and Beatty, W.W. (1978): Open-field and avoidance behavior after neostriatal lesions in male and female rats. *J. Comp. Physiol. Psychol.* 92:297-311.

Swanson, H.E. and van der Werff ten Bosch, J.J. (1964): The "early androgen" syndrome, its development and the response to hemi-spaying. *Acta Endocrinol.* 45:1-12.

Swanson, H.E. and van der Werff ten Bosch, J.J. (1965): The "early androgen" syndrome: Differences in response to pre-natal and post-natal administration of various doses of testosterone propionate in female and male rats. *Acta Endocrinol.* 47:37-50.

Swanson, H.H. (1966): Sex differences in behaviour of hamsters in open field and emergence tests: Effects of pre- and post-pubertal gonadectomy. *Anim. Behav.* 14:522-529.

Swanson, H.H. (1967): Alteration of sex-typical behaviour of hamsters in open field and emergence tests by neo-natal administration of androgen or estrogen. *Anim. Behav.* 15: 209-216.

Swanson, H.H. (1971): Determination of the sex role in hamsters by the action of sex hormones in infancy. *In: Influence of Hormones on the Nervous System.* Ford, D.H., ed. Basel: S. Karger, pp. 424-440.

Swanson, H.H. and Crossley, D.A. (1971): Sexual behaviour in the golden hamster and its modification by neonatal administration of testosterone propionate. *In: Hormones in Development.* Hamburgh, M. and Barrington, E.J., eds. New York: Appleton-Century-Crofts, pp. 677-687.

Taleisnik, S., Caligaris, L., and Astrada, J.J. (1969): Sex difference in the release of luteinizing hormone evoked by progesterone. *J. Endocrinol.* 44:313-321.

Tarttelin, M.F. and Gorski, R.A. (1973): The effects of ovarian steroids on food and water intake and body weight in the female rat. *Acta Endocrinol.* 72:551-568.

Tarttelin, M.F., Shryne, J.E., and Gorski, R.A. (1975): Patterns of body weight change in rats following neonatal hormone manipulation: a "critical period" for androgen-induced growth increases. *Acta Endocrinol.* 79:177-191.

Telegdy, G. and Stark, A. (1973): Effect of sexual steroids and androgen sterilization on avoidance and exploratory behavior in the rat. *Acta Physiol. Acad. Sci. Hung.* 43:55-63.

Thiessen, D.D. and Rice, M. (1976): Mammalian scent gland marking and social behavior. *Psychol. Bull.* 83:505-539.

Thiessen, D.D. and Yahr, P. (1970): Central control of territorial marking in the Mongolian gerbil. *Physiol. Behav.* 5:275-278.

Thomas, T.R. and Gerall, A.A. (1969): Dissociation of reproductive physiology and behavior induced by neonatal treatment with steroids. *Endocrinology* 85:781-784.

Thompson, M.L., McGill, T.E., McIntosh, S.M., and Manning, A. (1976): The effects of adrenalectomy on the sexual behavior of castrated and intact BDF_1 mice. *Anim. Behav.* 24:519-522.

Thorpe, W.H. (1958): The learning of song patterns by birds, with especial reference to the song of the chaffinch, *Fringilla coelebs. Ibis* 100:335-370.

Thorpe, W.H. and North, M.E.W. (1965): Origin and significance of the power of vocal imitation: with special reference to the antiphonal singing of birds. *Nature* 208:219-222.

Tiefer, L. (1970): Gonadal hormones and mating behavior in the adult golden hamster. *Horm. Behav.* 1:189-202.

Tinbergen, N. (1951): *The Study of Instinct.* Oxford: Clarendon Press.

Tinbergen, N. (1952): Derived activities: their causation, biological significance, origin and emancipation during evolution. *Quart. Rev. Biol.* 27:1-32.

Tinbergen, N. (1953): *The Herring Gull's World.* London: Collins.

Tinbergen, N. (1954): The origin and evolution of courtship and threat display. *In: Evolution as a Process.* Huxley, J.S., Hardy, A.C., and Ford, E.B., eds. London: Allen and Unwin, pp. 233-250.

Tinbergen, N. (1965): Some recent studies of the evolution of sexual behavior. *In: Sex and Behaviour.* Beach, F.A., ed. New York: John Wiley and Sons.

Toran-Allerand, C.D. (1976): Sex steroids and the development of the newborn mouse hypothalamus and preoptic area in vitro: implications for sexual differentiation. *Brain Res.* 106:407-412.

Toran-Allerand, C.D., Gerlach, J.L., and McEwen, B.S. (1978): Autoradiographic responsiveness in cultures of the hypothalamus/preoptic area. *In: Society for Neurosciences Abstracts, Vol. 4.* (Eighth Annual Meeting of the Society for Neuroscience, St. Louis, MO, Nov. 5-9, 1978.) P. 129.

Trampuž, V. (1968): Partial refractoriness to cortisone therapy in the adrenogenital syndrome. *In: Research on Steroids, Vol. III.* Cassano, C., et al., eds. Amsterdam: Elsevier/North-Holland Biomedical Press, P. 347.

Tryon, R.C. (1931): Studies in individual differences in maze ability: II. The determination of individual differences by age, weight, sex, and pigmentation. *J. Comp. Psychol.* 12:1-22.

Tuohimaa, P. and Johansson, R. (1971): Decreased estradiol binding in the uterus and anterior hypothalamus of androgenized female rats. *Endocrinology* 88:1159-1164.

Turkelson, C.M., Dunlap, J.L., MacPhee, A.A., and Gerall, A.A. (1977): Assay of perinatal testosterone and influence of anti-progesterone and theophylline on induction of sterility. *Life Sci.* 21:1149-1157.

Turner, J.W. (1975): Influence of neonatal androgen on the display of territorial marking in the gerbil. *Physiol. Behav.* 15:265-270.

Uriel, J. and de Nechaud, B. (1973): An outline of the physiopathology of rat alpha-fetoprotein. *In: Alpha-Fetoprotein and Hepatoma.* Hirari, H. and Miyaji, T., eds. Baltimore: University Park Press, pp. 35-47.

Uriel, J., de Nechaud, B., and Dupiers, M. (1972): Estrogen-binding properties of rat, mouse, and man fetospecific serum proteins. Demonstration by immuno-autoradiographic methods. *Biochem. Biophys. Res. Commun.* 46:1175-1180.

Vaccari, A., Brotman, S., Cimino, J., and Timiras, P. (1977): Sex differentiation of neurotransmitter enzymes in central and peripheral nervous systems. *Brain Res.* 132:176-185.

Vale, J.R., Ray, D., and Vale, C.A. (1972): The interaction of genotype and exogenous neonatal androgen: agonistic behavior in female mice. *Behav. Biol.* 7:321-334.

Valenstein, E.S. (1968): Steroid hormones and the neuropsychology of development. *In: The Neuropsychology of Development.* Isacsson, R.L., ed. New York: John Wiley and Sons, Inc., pp. 1-39.

Valenstein, E.S., Cox, V.C., and Kakolewski, J.W. (1969): Sex differences in hyperphagia and body weight following hypothalamic damage. *Ann. N.Y. Acad. Sci.* 157:1030-1048.

Valenstein, E.S., Kakolewski, J.W., and Cox, V.C. (1967): Sex differences in taste preference for glucose and saccharin solutions. *Science* 156:942-943.

van der Schoot, P., van der Vaart, P.D.M., and Vreebury, J.T.M. (1976): Masculinization in male rats is inhibited by neonatal injections of dihydrotestosterone. *J. Reprod. Fertil.* 48:385-387.

Verhoeven, G. and Wilson, J.D. (1976): Cytosol androgen binding in submandibular gland and kidney of the normal mouse and the mouse with testicular feminization. *Endocrinology* 99:79-92.

Verner, J. and Engelsen, G.H. (1970): Territories, multiple nest building, and polygyny in the long-billed marsh wren. *Auk* 87:557-567.

Vertes, M. and King, R.J.B. (1971): The mechanism of oestradiol binding in rat hypothalamus: effect of androgenization. *Endocrinology* 51:271-282.

Veyssi, G., Berger, M., Jean-Faucher, C.H., de Turckheim, M., and Jean, C.L. (1975): Radioimmunoassay of testosterone in late fetal and newborn rabbit plasma, gonads and adrenal glands. *Arch. Int. Physiol. Biochim.* 83:667-682.

Vilberg, T.R. and Beatty, W.W. (1975): Behavioral changes following VMH lesions in rats with controlled insulin levels. *Pharmacol. Biochem. Behav.* 3:377-384.

Vito, C.C. and Fox, T.O. (1977): Embryonic estradiol receptors from mouse and rat brain. *In: Society for Neuroscience Abstracts, Vol. III.* (Seventh Annual Meeting of the Society for Neuroscience, Anaheim, CA, Nov. 6-10, 1977.) P. 359.

Vito, C.C. and Fox, T.O. (1979): Embryonic rodent brain contains estrogen receptors. *Science* 204:517-519.

vom Saal, F.S. and Bronson, F.H. (1978): In utero proximity of female mouse fetuses to males: effect on reproductive performance during later life. *Biol. Reprod.* 19:842-853.

Vreeburg, J.T.M., van der Vaart, P.D.M., and van der Schoot, P. (1977): Prevention of central defeminization but not masculinization in male rats by inhibition neonatally of oestrogen biosynthesis. *J. Endocrinol.* 74:375-382.

Wade, G.N. (1976): Sex hormones, regulatory behaviors, and body weight. *In: Advances in the Study of Behavior, Vol. 6.* Rosenblatt, J.S., Hinde, R.A., Shaw, E., and Beer, C.G., eds. New York: Academic Press, pp. 201-279.

Wade, G.N. and Zucker, I. (1969): Taste preferences of female rats: Modification by neonatal hormones, food deprivation, and prior experience. *Physiol. Behav.* 4:935-943.

Wade, G.N. and Zucker, I. (1970a) Hormonal modulation of responsiveness to an aversive taste stimulus in rats. *Physiol. Behav.* 5:269-273.

Wade, G.N. and Zucker, I. (1970b): Modulation of food intake and locomotor activity in female rats by diencephalic hormone implants. *J. Comp. Physiol. Psychol.* 72:328-336.

Wagner, J.W., Erwin, W., and Critchlow, V. (1966): Androgen sterilization produced by intracerebral implants of testosterone in neonatal female rats. *Endocrinology* 79:1135-1142.

Wallen, K., Goy, R.W., and Phoenix, C.H. (1975): Inhibitory actions of progesterone on hormonal induction of estrus in female guinea pigs. *Horm. Behav.* 6:127-138.

Wallis, C.J. and Luttge, W.G. (1975): Maintenance of male sexual behaviour by combined treatment with oestrogen and dihydrotestosterone in CD-1 mice. *J. Endocrinol.* 66:257-262.

Walsh, P.C., Madden, J.D., Harrod, M.J., Goldstein, J.L., MacDonald, P.C., and Wilson, J.D. (1974): Familial incomplete male pseudohermaphroditism, Type 2. Decreased dihydrotestosterone formation in pseudovaginal perineoscrotal hypospadias. *New Eng. J. Med.* 291: 944-949.

Walsh, P.C. and Wilson, J.D. (1976): The induction of prostatic hypertrophy in the dog with androstanediol. *J. Clin. Invest.* 57:1093-1097.

Ward, I.L. (1969): Differential effect of pre- and postnatal androgen on the sexual behavior of intact and spayed female rats. *Horm. Behav.* 1:25-36.

Ward, I.L. (1972): Female sexual behavior in male rats treated prenatally with an anti-androgen. *Physiol. Behav.* 8:53-56.

Ward, I.L. (1974): Sexual behavior differentiation: prenatal hormonal and environmental control. *In: Sex Differences in Behavior.* Friedman, R.C., Richart, R.M., and Vande Wiele, R.L., eds. New York: John Wiley and Sons, Inc., pp. 3-17.

Ward, I.L. and Renz, F.J. (1972): Consequences of perinatal hormone manipulation on the adult sexual behavior of female rats. *J. Comp. Physiol. Psychol.* 78:349-355.

Ward, I.L. and Weisz, J. (1977): The role of testosterone in sexual behavior differentiation of male and female rats. Presented at the 85th Annual Convention of the American Psychological Association, San Francisco, August, 1977.

Warne, G.L., Faiman, C., Reyes, F.I., and Winter, J.S.D. (1977): Studies on human sexual development. V. Concentrations of testosterone, 17-hydroxyprogesterone and progesterone in human aminiotic fluid throughout gestation. *J. Clin. Endocrinol. Metab.* 44:934-938.

Warren, D.W., Haltmeyer, G.C., and Eik-Ness, K.B. (1973): Testosterone in the fetal rat testis. *Biol. Reprod.* 8:560-565.

Warren, D.W., Haltmeyer, G.C., and Eik-Ness, K.B. (1975): The effect of gonadotrophins on fetal and neonatal rat testis. *Endocrinology* 96:1226-1229.

Washburn, S.L. and Dolhinow, P., eds. (1972): *Perspectives on Human Evolution, Vol. 2.* New York: Holt, Rinehart and Winston.

Weisz, J. and Gibbs, C. (1974a): Conversion of testosterone and androstenedione to estrogens *in vitro* by the brain of female rats. *Endocrinology* 94:616-620.

Weisz, J. and Gibbs, C. (1974b): Metabolites of testosterone in the brain of the newborn female rat after an injection of tritiated testosterone. *Neuroendocrinology* 14:72-86.

Weisz, J., O'Brien, L.V., and Lloyd, T. (1978): Methylation of a partially purified preparation of bovine pineal hydroxy-indol-O-methyltransferase. *Endocrinology* 102:330-333.

Weisz, J. and Ward, I.L. (1979): Plasma testosterone and progesterone titers of pregnant rats, male and female fetuses and neonatal offsprings. *Endocrinology* (In press)

Weller, M.W. (1967): Notes on some marsh birds of Cape San Antonio, Argentina. *Ibis* 109: 391-411.

Westley, B.R. and Salaman, D.F. (1975): Incorporation of ^{3}H-uridine into RNA in the hypothalamus of the neonatal rat. *J. Endocrinol.* 65:58P-

Westley, B.R. Salaman, D.F. (1976): Role of oestrogen receptor in androgen-induced sexual differentiation of the brain. *Nature* 262:407-408.

Westley, B.R. and Salaman, D.F. (1977): Nuclear binding of the oestrogen receptor of neonatal rat brain after injection of oestrogens and androgens; localization and sex differences. *Brain Res.* 119:375-388.

Whalen, R.E. and DeBold, J.F. (1974): Comparative effectiveness of testosterone, androstenedione and dihydrotestosterone in maintaining mating behavior in the castrated male hamster. *Endocrinology* 95:1674-1675.

Whalen, R.E. and Edwards, D.A. (1967): Hormonal determinants of the development of masculine behavior in male and female rats. *Anat. Rec.* 157:173-180.

Whalen, R.E., Edwards, D.A., Luttge, W.G., and Robertson, R.T. (1969): Early androgen treatment and male sexual behavior in female rats. *Physiol. Behav.* 4:33-39.

Whalen, R.E. and Luttge, W.G. (1971): Testosterone, androstenedione, and dihydrotestosterone: effects on mating behavior of male rats. *Horm. Behav.* 2:117-125.

Whalen, R.E., Luttge, W.G., and Gorzalka, B.B. (1971): Neonatal androgenization and the development of estrogen responsivity in male and female rats. *Horm. Behav.* 2:83-90.

Whalen, R.E. and Nadler, R.D. (1963): Suppression of the development of female mating behavior by estrogen administration in infancy. *Science* 14:273-274.

Whalen, R.E. and Rezek, D.L. (1974): Inhibition of lordosis in female rats by subcutaneous implants of testosterone, androstenedione, or dihydrotestosterone in infancy. *Horm. Behav.* 5:125-128.

Whiting, B.B., ed. (1963): *Six Cultures: Studies of Child Rearing.* New York: John Wiley and Sons, Inc.

Whiting, B.B. and Whiting, J.W.M. (1974): *Children of Six Cultures: a Psycho-Cultural Analysis.* Cambridge, Mass.: Harvard University Press.

Whitsett, J.M., Bronson, F.H., Peters, P.J., and Hamilton, T.H. (1972): Neonatal organization of aggression in mice: Correlation of critical period with uptake of hormone. *Horm. Behav.* 3:11-21.

Whitsett, J.M., Irvin, E.W., Edens, F.W., and Thaxton, J.P. (1977): Demasculinization of male Japanese quail by prenatal estrogen treatment. *Horm. Behav.* 8:254-263.

Whitsett, J.M. and Vandenbergh, J.C. (1975): Influence of testosterone propionate administered neonatally on puberty and bisexual behavior in female hamsters. *J. Comp. Physiol. Psychol.* 88:248-255.

Wickler, W. (1967): Socio-sexual signals and their intra-specific imitation among primates. *In: Primate Ethology.* Morris, D., ed. Chicago: Aldine Publishing Co., pp. 69-147.

Wieland, S.J. and Fox, T.O. (1976): DNA affinity separates androgen and estrogen binding activity: study of residual androgen binding macromolecules in *Tfm* mutant mouse brain. *In: Neuroscience Abstracts, Vol.* II. (Sixth Annual Meeting of the Society for Neuroscience, Toronto, Canada, Nov. 7-11, 1976.) P. 661.

Wieland, S.J., Fox, T.O., and Savakis, C. (1978): DNA-binding of androgen and estrogen receptors from mouse brain: behavior of residual androgen receptor from *Tfm* mutant. *Brain Res.* 140:159-164.

Wiley, R.H. (1971): Song groups in a singing assembly of little hermits. Condor 73:28-35.

Wiley, R.H. (1973): Territoriality and non-random mating in sage grouse, *Centrocercus urophasianus. Anim. Behav.* 6:85-169.

Wiley, R.H. (1974): Evolution of social organization and life-history patterns among grouse. *Quart. Rev. Biol.* 49:201-227.

Williams, J.T. and North, RA (1979): Effects of endorphins on single myenteric neurons. *Brain Res.* (In press)

Willier, B.H. (1942): Hormonal control of embryonic differentiation in birds. *Cold Spring Harbor Symp. Quant. Biol.* 10:135-144.

Wilson, J.D. (1976a): Metabolism of testicular androgens. *In: Handbook of Physiology, Section 7: Endocrinology. Vol. 5. Male Reproductive System.* Greep, R.O. and Astwood, E.B., eds. Baltimore: Williams and Wilkins, pp. 491-508.

Wilson, J.D. (1976b): The use of genetic disorders for the analysis of sexual development. *Andrologia* (Suppl. 1): 8:35-42.

Wilson, J.D. and Gloyna, R.E. (1970): The intranuclear metabolism of testosterone in the accessory organs of reproduction. *Rec. Prog. Horm. Res.* 26:309-336.

Wilson, J.D. and Goldstein, J.L. (1975): Classification of hereditary disorders of sexual development. *Birth Defects:* Original Article Series, Vol. XI, No. 4, pp. 1-16.

Wilson, J.D., Harrod, M.J., Goldstein, J.L., Hensell, D.L., and MacDonald, P.C. (1974): Familial incomplete male pseudohermaphroditism, Type 1. Evidence for androgen resistance and variable clinical manifestations in a family with the Reifenstein Syndrome. *New Eng. J. Med.* 290:1097-1103.

Wilson, J.D. and Lasnitzki, I. (1971): Dihydrotestosterone formation in fetal tissues of the rabbit and rat. *Endocrinology* 89:659-668.

Wilson, J.D. and Siiteri, P.K. (1973): Developmental pattern of testosterone synthesis in the fetal gonad of the rabbit. *Endocrinology* 92:1182-1191.

Wise, S.P., Jones, E.G., and Berman, N. (1978): Direction and specificity of axonal and transcellular transport of nucleosides. *Brain Res.* 139:197-217.

Witschi, E. (1935): Die Amphisexualität der embryonalen Keimdrüsen des Haussperlings *Passer domesticus* (Linnaeus). *Biol. Zentralbl.* 55:168-174.

Witschi, E. (1961): Sex and secondary sexual characters. *In: Biology and Comparative Physiology of Birds, Vol. 2.* Marshal, A.J., ed. New York: Academic Press, pp. 115-168.

Wolff, Em. (1950): La différenciation sexuelle normale et le conditionnement hormonal des caractères sexuels somatiques précoces, tubercule génital et syrinx, chez l'embryon de Canard. *Bull. Biol. France et Belg.* 84:119-193.

Wolff, Et. (1950): Le rôle des hormones embryonnaires dans la différenciation sexuelle des oiseaux. *Arch. Anat. Microscop. Morphol. Exp.* 39:426-450.

Wolff, Et. (1952): La culture d'organes embryonnaires *in vitro. Rev. Sci.* 90:189-198.

Wolff, Et. and Wolff, Em. (1949): Application de la méthode de castration à l'embryon de canard: sur deux tests de l' activité précoce des gonades embryonnaires, la syrinx et le tubercule génital. *C.R. Acad. Soc. B* 143:529-531.

Wood, J.D. and Mayer, C.J. (1978a): Intracellular study of electrical behavior in tonic type myenteric neurons of guinea pig small bowel. *Fed. Proc.* 37:227. (Abstr.)

Wood, J.D. and Mayer, C.J. (1978b): Functional significance of slow EPSP in myenteric ganglion cells. *In: Neuroscience Abstracts, Vol. 4.* (Eighth Annual Meeting of the Society for Neuroscience, St. Louis, MO, Nov. 5-9, 1978.) P. 586.

Wood, J.D. and Mayer, C.J. (1979a): Intracellular study of tonic-type enteric neurons in guinea pig small intestine. *J. Neurophysiol.* 42:569-581.

Wood, J.D. and Mayer, C.J. (1979b): Serotonergic activation of tonic-type enteric neurons in guinea-pig small bowel. *J. Neurophysiol.* 42:582-593.

Woolsey, S.H. (1977): Pied Piper politics and the child-care debate. *Daedalus* 106:127-146.

Wright, P. and Turner, C. (1973): Sex differences in body weight following gonadectomy and goldthioglucose injections in mice. *Physiol. Behav.* 11:155-159.

Yahr, P., Coquelin, A., Martin, A., and Scouten, C.W. (1977): Effects of castration on aggression between male Mongolian gerbils. *Behav. Biol.* 19:189-205.

Yalom, J.D., Green, R., and Fisk, N. (1973): Prenatal exposure to female hormones: Effect on psychosexual development in boys. *Arch. Gen. Psychiatry* 28:554-561.

Yamamoto, T.O. and Kajishima, T. (1968): Sex hormone induction of sex reversal in the goldfish and evidence for male heterogamety. *J. Exp. Zool.* 168:215-221.

Yoshimura, F., Harumiya, K., and Kiyam, H. (1970): Light and electron microscopic studies of the cytogenesis of anterior pituitary cells in perinatal rats in reference to the development of target organs. *Arch. Histol. Jap.* 31:333-369.

Young, W.C., Goy, R.W., and Phoenix, C.H. (1964): Hormones and sexual behavior. Broad relationships exist between the gonadal hormones and behavior. *Science* 143:212-218.

Zadina, J. (1977): The effect of neonatal EB and TP on the development of male reproductive tissues and behavior. Master's Thesis, Tulane University, New Orleans, LA.

Zadina, J.E., Dunlap, J.L., and Gerall, A.A. (1979): Modifications induced by neonatal steroids in reproductive organs and behavior of male rats. *J. Comp. Physiol. Psychol.* 93:314-322.

Zimmerman, H. and Whittaker, V.P. (1974): Effect of electrical stimulation in the yield and composition of synaptic vesicles from the cholinergic synapses of the electric organ of *Torpedo:* a combined biochemical, electrophysiological and morphological study. *J. Neurochem.* 22:435-450.

Zondek, T., Mansfield, M.D., and Zondek, L.H. (1977): Amniotic fluid testosterone and fetal sex determination in the first half of pregnancy. *Br. J. Obstet. Gynaecol.* 84:714-716.

Zucker, I. (1969): Hormonal determinants of sex differences in saccharin preference, food intake, and body weight. *Physiol. Behav.* 4:595-602.

Zucker, I. (1972): Body weight and age as factors determining estrogen responsiveness in the rat feeding system. *Behav. Biol.* 7:527-542.

Zucker, I., Wade, G.N., and Ziegler, R. (1972): Sexual and hormonal influences on eating, taste preferences, and body weight of hamsters. *Physiol. Behav.* 8:101-111.

Zussman, J.U., Zussman, P.P., and Dalton, K. (1975): Post-pubertal effects of prenatal administration of progesterone. Paper presented at a meeting of the Society for Research in Child Development, Denver, CO.

INDEX